FIFTY MILES AT A BREATH

ONCE UPON A VET SCHOOL: VET SCHOOL 24/7

LIZZI TREMAYNE

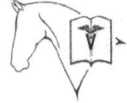

New Zealand and United States Copyright 2017 by Lizzi Tremayne

All rights reserved. No part of this publication may be reproduced, distributed or transmitted in any form or by any means, without prior written permission.

Lizzi Tremayne / Blue Mist Publishing

Franklin Road, RD 2

Waihi, New Zealand 3682

www.lizzitremayne.com

Publisher's Note: This is a work of fiction. Names, characters, places, and incidents are a product of the author's imagination. Locales and public names are sometimes used for atmospheric purposes. Any resemblance to actual people, living or dead, or to businesses, companies, events, institutions, or locales is completely coincidental.

Cover design and photos by Lizzi Tremayne. Photo credits to Canva (sunset) and Kirsten Petersen (endurance race), & Lizzi Tremayne (dogs)

Author photo credit to Kajai@gmail.com

Formatting and artwork by Lizzi Tremayne

Previously published with Authors of Main Street in Anthology: Summer Romance on Main Street 2018

From the Vet School 24/7 sequence of the **Once Upon a Vet School** series

Fifty Miles at a Breath/Lizzi Tremayne 1st Edition 2018 11 11

Printed in New Zealand and United States of America

Draft2Digital Paperback Edition 2019 06 13-V8

ISBN 978-0-9951157-9-8

DEDICATED TO

To Muriel Eston and Trudy Petersen
My grandmother and step-grandmother, and to all those other breast cancer warriors who held up their heads and fought valiantly to the end.

We will remember you.

~ ~ ~ ~ ~

~ *to Nonna Trudy:* I loved the festive, elegant holidays you created; my favorite stable play place; your lovely mare Tilla; the keen polo ponies and endurance horses; and your magnificent home. While I may have worn drab colors next to your Swiss butterfly brilliance, the autumn shades were my colors. I remember with pleasure the day you finally recognized it too—it made such a difference to us both. I'm so glad you finished the Tevis and earned that buckle, which you wore so proudly.

~ *to Ma Muriel,* from "Miss Clean 1972": I actually scrub up okay, you'd be pleased to know. Thank you for: Easter egg hunts in you massive front yard; swimming in your pool overlooking the College of Notre Dame; letting this little three-year-old make biscuits in (all over) your kitchen while wearing my Sunday best; your splendid yolkies and waddies; potato latkas; bagels and lox with red onions; the biggest thanksgiving turkeys I've ever seen to this day; and the back half of my first pony ("The half that doesn't eat," you said.); but especially, your love.

Lena finished this race for both of you.

With all my love, forever.

L-

CONTENTS

Books by Lizzi Tremayne	vii
Praise for Lizzi Tremayne	ix
Chapter 1	1
Chapter 2	13
Chapter 3	21
Chapter 4	31
Chapter 5	41
Chapter 6	51
Chapter 7	61
Chapter 8	71
Chapter 9	83
Chapter 10	93
Chapter 11	105
Chapter 12	115
Chapter 13	125
Chapter 14	135
Chapter 15	149
Chapter 16	161
Chapter 17	173
Chapter 18	181
Chapter 19	191
Chapter 20	201
Chapter 21	211
Chapter 22	221
Find Books	233
Books by the Author	235
Author's Notes	245
Recipe: Cottage Cheese Pancakes	247
About the Author	249

Connect with Lizzi	251
Acknowledgments	253
Excerpt from A Long Trail Rolling	255
Excerpt from Tatiana	263

BOOKS BY LIZZI TREMAYNE

The Long Trails Series
A Long Trail Rolling (Book One)
The Hills of Gold Unchanging (Book Two)
A Sea of Green Unfolding (Book Three)

Multi-Series Samplers
Lizzi Tremayne First Chapter Sampler

The Once Upon a Vet School Series
~Vet School 24/7~
Fifty Miles at a Breath
Lena Takes a Foal
~Practice Time~
Greener Pastures Calling

Boxed sets with Authors of Main Street
Christmas Babies on Main Street
Summer Romance on Main Street
Christmas Wishes on Main Street

Boxed sets with Bluestocking Belles
Follow Your Star Home

Sign up for Lizzi's VIP Readers Club to hear about new releases and specials, plus get your free sampler gift here:

www.lizzitremayne.com/VIP50

PRAISE FOR LIZZI TREMAYNE

With her debut novel, **A Long Trail Rolling,** *Lizzi was:*

Winner 2016 True West Magazine
Best Western Romance
Winner 2015 RWNZ Koru Award
Finalist 2015 Best Indie Book Award
Winner 2014 RWNZ Pacific Hearts Award
Finalist 2013 RWNZ Great Beginnings

"vivid, light and fast-paced… a ripping good read. "
–Deborah Challinor, number one bestselling author and historian

"An authentic, emotional story of one woman's fight for survival in an unforgiving landscape."
–Leeanna Morgan, USA Today bestselling author

"An impressive debut…a romance, a western, and an adventure story, all rolled up into a compelling read."
–Booksellers NZ

The Hills of Gold Unchanging:
"The pace is fast, there's plenty of action and adventure and a few twists I didn't see coming. Good characters plus excellent history equals a great read."
—*Deborah Challinor, number one bestselling author and historian*

"...superb storytelling."
—*Judy Knighton, editor*

"I particularly liked the attention to historical detail. This is an author who does her homework, and it shows... a cracking good yarn."
—*Shelagh Merlin, NetGalley Reviewer*

A Sea of Green Unfolding:
"the historical research is excellent...well-integrated into the narrative."
—*Deborah Challinor, number one bestselling author and historian*

"A lovely combination of historical accuracy and adventure... [a] beautifully researched and engrossing story."
—*Shelagh Merlin, NetGalley reviewer*

"Loved this book. The characters draw you in on a story filled with interest and suspense."
—*Kate Le Petit*

Fifty Miles at a Breath
"Lizzi Tremayne is a born storyteller. The...characters... [are] three dimensional and you can feel Lena and Blake's emotions."
—*Lori Dykes*

"a wonderful series about the path to becoming a veterinarian, the love of horses and sweet romance. Lena and Blake will grab your heart."
—Teri Donaldson

Lena Takes a Foal

"This book is for anyone with a passion for horses… or anyone who loves a story about strong, independent young women finding love!"
—Stacey

"The story… displays Lizzi Tremayne's ability to develop strong characters… with a nice strong black moment to challenge our heroine and prove her worth."
—Shelagh Merlin, NetGalley Reviewer

"…the perfect blend of sweet romance, horses and real emotions with fascinating information woven in about the medical care of horses."
—Teri Donaldson

"As I turned the last page I cannot stop smiling! I look forward to more in this series and from this author!!!"
—Lori Dykes

1

1986 Southern California

"You'll regret you refused me," Gareth Barnett-Payne growled, reaching for me, but I spun and ran until my legs—

"Lena... Lena." Raywyn, the head veterinary technician, waved her hand before my eyes.

I blinked, shaking my head and willing my heart to stop pounding in my chest.

"Are you okay?" Her brows knitted together.

I gripped the edge of the desk before me. "Yes, fine," I mumbled, wondering how anyone could be so vicious. "So"— I swallowed hard and dragged myself back to today— "what's the surgery schedule for tomorrow, Ray?"

She looked at me sideways, then turned to the schedule before her.

I took a deep breath and let it out slowly, trying to release the tension stacked up from three weeks of flea allergy dermatitis, hotspots, anal glands and catfight abscesses.

Through those stinking hot Santa Barbara summer days, I yearned for the touch of a velvet nose, the solid muscle and bone, and the scent of a horse. *Any* horse. It wouldn't be much longer before I could go home to my own roan. I bit my lip and scanned the small animal clinic, my eyes and nose running as freely as they'd been since the moment I first walked in through the practice doorway. Cat allergy in a vet—great. Thank god I was going to be an equine vet.

"Let's see..." Ray's finger ran down the page. "Two dogs spays, a cruciate surgery, four cat neuters, and... hmmm... I can't read it. I'll need to ask Dr. Franco." She flashed a grin at me. "With your handwriting, you should make a fantastic veterinarian, too. I can't read a thing you write."

"I really do try," I said, with a rueful grin.

"Could have fooled me."

"Not too many cats for tomorrow, then," I sighed, "that's a good thing."

"We don't have many appointments, so Dr. Franco will be free to supervise and you should be able to do most of the surgeries."

"I'm pretty lucky." I nodded. "I get to do so much surgery here. I've been speaking with some of my classmates. They just don't get the opportunities I've been handed. I'll be forever grateful to you and Dr. Franco for that. I'm going to be a horse vet, but I'm sure there'll still be other animals in my life."

Ray looked at me, brows narrowed, until I began to squirm with an overwhelming urge to cover myself. "What?"

"It's a man, isn't it?"

I gritted my teeth and held my breath. "Maybe."

"No maybe about it. Who is he?"

"Some creep with a control fetish."

Ray blinked and shook her head. "Tell me he isn't your problem anymore."

"He's not my problem anymore."

"Truth?"

I nodded. "Never was, much, though he encouraged the idea… rather forcefully."

"You need to come out with us to a few clubs tomorrow night. Just the girls."

"I'd rather stay away from men, but thanks all the same."

Ray's smile faded. "It'll be fun, Lena. It's a group of women. We'll dance, have a blast, and go home. Alone. Can you think about it?" Her smile was hopeful.

"I'll think about it," I said, biting my lip. "Can I tell you tomorrow?"

"Sure, but we'd love to have you along."

"I don't know… I'm truly over men," I swallowed hard. "They're just not worth the angst."

"All you have to do is come out with us. You don't even need to dance with them. You can dance with the rest of the girls."

I was far from certain, but I had no other plans for my hot Friday night. "Okay," I finally said.

THE ELECTRONIC MUSIC throbbing across the dance floor jangled in my head. It was so loud, my heart thumped in shock along with the beat. With a deep breath, I forced my butt to stay on the barstool. And tried to smile. And look pleasant. Hard when everything about the place made me want to run screaming out the door. The men either plastic and young in their shiny, synthetic shi—

"Aren't you glad you came with us, now?" Ray's voice cut into my thoughts during a momentary lull in the noise.

I bit my cheek and nodded. No use wrecking her night, too. There certainly wasn't anyone here with whom I'd want to wake up, much less spend the rest of my life. Maybe I was just too serious.

"That guy"—Ray nodded her chin—"the one who looks like he never leaves the beach, has been eyeing you up for the past half hour. Why don't you go put him out of his misery?"

I rolled my eyes as the music started pounding again. "Come on, Ray, you know I can't shoot guys in here," I shouted over the music and smirked. "Someone might object."

Ray closed her eyes and shook her head. "You really are a tough case, aren't you?" she yelled back.

"Okay, I'll go. I don't imagine he knows how to dance Western Swing," I said into her ear as I hopped from my perch.

"You go girl!" Ray barked, her eyes twinkling.

Mr. Lifeguard may have been eyeing me up, but he looked ready to bolt at my approach.

"Hi, my friend thought I should come ask you to dance."

"Hello," he said with a heavy accent and I blinked.

"A Danish hello?" A smile cracked my visage.

This *could be interesting*.

His rabbit-in-the-headlights look dissolved and he laughed.

"*Hvordan har due de?*" he said, in my mother's native language.

"*Fint tak*," I replied. That made me smile. My mother would be pleased.

He started off on a stream of rapid-fire *dansk*, and with a laugh, I put a hand on his arm to stop him.

"Whoa there. You've already heard most of my Danish. From my mom, I learned hello, thank you, you're welcome, and stand up. Baby words."

His smile melted and he bit his lip.

"It's okay," I smiled. "Want to dance?"

"*Tak*, thank you. That, I would love," he said, as he put a hand on the small of my back and guided me to the crowded dance floor.

"You wouldn't know how to dance properly, would you?"

With a smile that lit the whole room, he took my hand and whirled me around the floor. The man could dance—and I was thankful once again for my many years of Latin and ballroom lessons. I never knew when they'd come in handy, like now.

"What are you doing so far from home?" I asked, after we'd been dancing for what seemed like hours.

"I've been at University here, studying marine biology."

"Really?" So, the lifeguard guess was close. "I almost did that. I love to dive—I started when I was an undergraduate here," I shouted, "but I'm in veterinary school up north now. Maybe we could go for a dive before I have to go home."

"I would love to"—he bit his lip, his brow furrowed—"but I fly back to *Danmark* tomorrow morning. I wish we'd met sooner." He genuinely looked wistful and my heart twinged at the thought of the friendship we might have had.

"Believe me when I say I'm gutted to hear you're leaving." That'd be right. I finally meet someone with the same interests… and he's heading halfway around the world the next day.

"Gutted?"

"Sorry, very sorry." My mouth twisted.

"Me too," said the Viking. He took my hand and made a little bow over it, then he kissed it. I had to take a deep breath and lock my knees to keep from melting. I love Europeans.

"It seems your friends are ready to leave." He nodded at Ray's table full of women. They looked at us over their empty glasses, purses slung over their shoulders. "*Mange tusind tak*, and goodbye for now," he said, as he turned away toward his own friends.

Many thousand thanks…

My heart sinking, I rejoined Ray and her friends as they walked out the door.

Outside on the street, Ray and I split from her friends and turned toward our apartment over the clinic. Ray stared at the retreating back of the blonde Viking as he and his friends headed away from us and tripped over a crack in the pavement. She recovered and turned back to me. Her mouth twitched in the light of the streetlamp. "Well, you've certainly found yourself a live one," she said, with a wink. "When will you see him again?"

I snorted. "Probably never. He flies home to Denmark tomorrow."

Ray's face fell. "You can't be serious."

"Story of my life." I nodded. "Told you it's not worth it,"—I couldn't repress a smile—"but the dancing was spectacular."

"You two were awesome out there."

"It was all him. I just followed."

"Could have fooled me," Ray muttered.

"Truth be told, it's easier, or safer, anyway, than dancing Western Swing, where the only rules are to try to stay on your feet while they fling you around. It's fun, but Jesper's dancing was… so much more subtle. It was easy, like… like… *dancing*." I beamed at my friend. "Thank you for dragging me along. I really enjoyed myself."

"You at least have each other's contacts, right?"

My mouth dropped open and nothing came out.

"I can see," Ray sighed, "I'll need to take you under my wing. You clearly lack training."

We both laughed, but mine was a bit self-conscious.

"I'll be okay." I gave her a half smile. "My focus needs to be veterinary school now. I really don't have the time or the energy for anything other than that. The next two years are going to be hard enough just taking care of me and my animals, without worrying about the ups and downs of a relationship."

"I see," Ray said, though she looked like she did no such thing.

"It's really true," I said firmly, wrapped an arm around Ray's shoulders, and gave her a squeeze. "I have friends like you. What more could a vet student want?"

"I guess you're right, and you have your precious horse waiting for you back at home." Ray stopped dead and stared at me. "Oh my god, horse...." She slapped her palm to her forehead and jerked her head toward me. "How could I forget about you?"

"Pardon?"

"A vet tech friend of mine asked me last week if I knew anyone who could help at an endurance ride next weekend."

"Like a *horse* endurance ride?" I goggled at her.

"No, you goof, they're racing *penguins*. Of course, it's a horse endurance ride." Ray's eyes sparkled. She'd grown up with horses, but with her head tech position at the clinic, she didn't have time for them now.

"Where do I sign?"

"Have you ever helped at an endurance ride?"

"I've been on the 'P & R Team' at the vet school and my family's done endurance since before I was born—I've been on my family's Tevis Cup crew since before I could walk."

"Boy, am I glad to hear that." Ray let out a breath and shook her head. "Sarah's desperate for some helpers." She turned to me, brow furrowed. "What's a P & R team?"

"P for pulse, R for respiration. It's a team of vet students that helps at local endurance rides by taking heart rates and respiratory rates on the horses before they go on to the vets at the control checks. It frees the vets up to focus on lameness and metabolic problems."

"Oh, of course."

"Where is it?" A tingle of excitement ran up my back.

"It's at Los Lomitos, about an hour and a half from here. I'll make you a deal: if you go help Sarah, you can leave on Friday at noon and needn't be back at work until Tuesday morning—you can take some time for yourself up there."

The weight, the tension sliding from my shoulders made me want to dance the rest of the way home. I was grateful for the opportunity offered by this summer preceptorship, but I wasn't sure if I'd survive a whole two months down here, away from home and my animals, with only patient dogs and cats for company. Ray was offering me not only respite, but horses, too.

"Sweeten the deal," Ray said at my continued silence. "I'll send you with my tent, sleeping bag, and everything you'll need to camp in luxury. Including poison oak medication."

I laughed, afraid my cheeks might split from smiling so widely. "I'm in. You had me at hello."

IT WAS STILL early afternoon on Friday when I arrived at the endurance race campground and found Ray's friend Sarah, the ride manager.

I'd beamed at myself in the rearview mirror for most of the drive. Four days of horses, camping, and outdoor life after the desert of life in a city. I'd owe Ray forever.

The somewhat frazzled Sarah managed a welcoming smile for me. "There's nothing you need to do until later, Lena," she said, handing me a lanyard and passes. "Ray told me your history, and I can't say how glad I am to have a volunteer of your experience and training."

"Happy to help," I said. "I just want to touch some horses."

"Plenty of opportunity for that." Sarah's eyes twinkled.

"The P & R team briefing starts at 7 p.m. and there's another session afterward to practice taking pulse and respiratory rates. You wouldn't want to help with that, would you?"

"Of course," I said. "I'm at your disposal."

"I'd hoped you'd say that. Most of the team are experienced horse people, but only a few have taken vitals before."

"I'd be happy to help them." I smiled.

"Thanks so much." Sarah's eyes glinted. "Go ahead and set up your camp. There's a nice swimming hole in the creek, just down there," she pointed, "if you feel so inclined. I need to run," she said, as a man wearing an OFFICIAL badge touched her on the shoulder, an expectant look on his face. "I'll see you at dinner." Sarah and the man headed off at a trot.

As my meals were supplied by the ride management, setting up camp took only minutes and I was soon free to enjoy my afternoon.

A luxury I haven't had in long months.

Inside Ray's tent, I dropped my jeans and slipped into my shorts and bikini top, grabbed a towel, and headed for the proffered swimming hole. I hadn't gotten far when the throaty rumble of an Arabian caught my attention. He stared at me intently from his wooden tie stall and I approached him, looking around for someone connected to this magnificent creature, but no one was near. His blood bay coat gleamed over a faultlessly muscled body. He whickered again as I neared him. With his body carriage, he had to be a stallion, so I peeked under his belly. Yep, a stallion.

I reached out a hand to him and he lipped gently at my palm.

"Ooh, aren't you the most handsome man?" I murmured.

I jumped when he answered.

"Why, thank you," came a deep voice, tinged with humor.

I chuckled into the laughing gaze of the man who raised

himself from the ground behind the short wall at the stallion's feet. "I thought he answered me for a moment."

The man's face creased into deep laugh lines around his gorgeous blue eyes. He was as handsome as the horse, to be sure.

"He talks, this boy," he said, as he slid one arm over the bay's back and gave him a scratch on his withers, then stuck out his other hand. "Blake, Blake Sagan. Pleased to meet you."

I smiled and introduced myself. "Just admiring your stallion. He's a beaut."

"Thanks. He's pretty special. His name's Prince. Prince Witeż, after his grandfather. My pride and joy. Are you racing tomorrow?"

"Not this time. I'm here to help, P & R team."

"Ever been to an endurance ride before?" He looked sideways at me while he waited for my answer.

"Oh, a few. My grandfather's done the Tevis Cup numerous times, my mom and stepdad a few more, and I've done some shorter rides plus ride & ties. I usually get to crew, though."

"Ah," his eyes glinted, "you must be the vet student from Santa Barbara."

I blinked. News traveled fast.

"I knew Sarah was looking for helpers." He smiled. "Thanks for coming along."

"Glad to help. I was in serious need of a horse fix. I've been working in a small animal clinic this summer."

"Not keen on the smallies?"

"I love them, but my heart's with the horses."

"You off for a swim?" He nodded at my towel.

"Sure am. Sarah told me to go down by the bridge."

"It's a nice spot, but there's an even better one a little way upstream. I'm taking Prince down there for a swim shortly."

"I'll see you down there, then."

"Be there soon," he said, and waved at me as I walked away.

Blake's gaze—there was more light in that man's sparkling eyes then I'd seen in ages. I wondered what he did besides ride horses—with that quick, intelligent spark, it must be something special.

What can I be thinking?

The next two years are not about having more devastating relationships. It's time to finish my doctorate and establish my career.

I cannot go there.

I simply cannot.

2

The clip-clop of hooves on stones let me know Blake and Prince were finally here. I shaded my eyes against the sun, looked up the hill, and blinked.

Did the man have to look like that in a pair of swim trunks? Really?

You found the place, I see." Blake's honeyed voice slid over me as I lay back down in the sun, trying to ignore the bronzed god coming down the hill toward me. He negotiated the last steep portion of the bank and stood before me. We both turned back to watch the magnificent bay nimbly pick his way down the narrow trail.

The stallion practically dragged him straight into the water and Blake hopped up onto his back as the stallion waded in deeper, laughing as the horse struck out across the deep part of the river, swimming for the other side.

"Not many horses would do *that* by choice," I called out.

He's different, this guy," Blake said, his deep voice carrying across the water. He grabbed at the bay's mane as the horse shook the water out of his coat, nearly dropping him.

"He doesn't look scrawny, like most of the fit endurance

horses I've ever seen…" I hesitated, then cringed a bit as I continued. "Are you sure he's fit to race tomorrow?"

Most riders wouldn't appreciate a comment like that, but I was, frankly, concerned. The stallion looked ready to walk into the arena at the Arabian National Show or into a breeding shed, not race fifty miles over rough mountain trails.

"Vets!" He laughed. "They're always worried about that. I guarantee you, he'll be in the same condition at the end of the race. Better yet, I'll bet you a nice steak dinner that he'll finish in perfect health."

I glanced sideways at him. He was *not* helping my resolve. "I'll skip on the bet, thanks, but I can't wait to see him at the finish line."

"You're on." Blake slid from the horse's back. Holding the end of the stallion's long lead, he swam lazily back to where I sat on the bank.

His quick appraisal of me in my short jean cutoffs and a string bikini top couldn't truly be considered an ogle, but it was enough to warm my cheeks. Fair's fair. I'd done more at the sight of him while he was occupied clambering down the riverbank. Best get my head out of the gutter.

"Have you been in the water? Your hair's still dry."

"Thought I'd warm up first, after dipping my foot in." Under his frank perusal, I decided I was definitely warm enough to swim, stood up, and looked for a spot deep enough to dive in.

"Lost something?"

"No, I'm just a wimp about getting into cold water. Easiest if I dive in."

He cocked one brow at me and quirked his mustache. "I'm a bit of an all-in/all-out kind of guy, too. Dive in head first, usually."

I frowned, my heart clenching a bit. A shadow crossing his

face said he might be talking about more than hopping into a pool of water, too, but then it was gone.

I dived. And came up sputtering. The bay drank deep from the water two yards away, ears pricked, his liquid eyes gazing into mine. I glanced back at Blake.

"He's okay. Call him."

"Prince," I murmured.

He lifted his head, muzzle dripping water, and sniffed the air between us. The stallion seemed to come to a decision and strode through the water toward my outstretched hand, then came closer and lipped gently at my fingers. I scratched under his forelock, then atop his withers, while he preened. Prince took a sideways step closer, shook his head then reached around to nuzzle me.

"You can hop on and he'll bring you back. He won't mind." Blake chuckled. "You're his, now. He's a true man."

I hadn't swung up on a horse with such a round barrel in years, much less from a position knee-deep in water. Prince stood like a rock while I clambered on, then he carefully picked his way into the deep water and swam me back to Blake.

"This horse is magical," I breathed, stroking his sleek neck, then barely stayed on when he shook again. "What a shake!" I grinned. "Haven't had such a shaking since my first pony, 'Lady' used to try to lose me when I was little."

"Something else, isn't he?" Blake turned his gaze to the dripping stallion. "Never had a horse like him, and I've had some good ones."

"How long have you been riding endurance?" I slid to the ground and hugged the horse. "Thank you," I whispered into the stallion's mane, and stepped away.

"About ten years. Prince has been racing with me for the past four. He's unstoppable. Just have to be aware of who's around when you're riding a stallion."

"Have you always ridden stallions, then?"

"No, he's my first. I'm just used to having to be aware of everything around me, anyway, because of my work."

"Work?"

He sighed. "I'm a pilot."

"Ah." His can-do attitude and watchfulness fit with that. I waited for elaboration, but there was none. "You fly for…?" I ventured, looking at him sideways.

"Short-haul commuters for Western Sky, out of Bakersfield. Not exciting, but it pays the bills."

"Any flying"—I winked at him over Prince's back—"is exciting."

A reluctant smile spread slowly over his face. "I guess so."

"What's wrong with being a pilot?" I stared at him. "It sounds like one of the best jobs in the world, after being a vet."

"Well, there is that, but… people seem…" he considered for a moment, "to think you're a good catch. Attracts the wrong sort of women. The money-grubbing kind."

"Really?" I'd never considered anything of the sort.

"Must be. I'm done with that."

"Me, too." Our eyes met, and we smiled, then I looked away for a moment. "My goals right now"—I turned back to him—"are finishing my degree and building the next step of my career."

"Good plan." He nodded. "Do you have any duties here before tomorrow morning?"

I told him, and he nodded.

"Prince and I are going for a little ride to loosen up, but we'll be back soon. If you'd like, I'll introduce you to some people tonight before dinner.

"I'd like that," I said, and meant it. I enjoyed talking with him… more than I should, probably.

"Come on by the truck when you're ready," he said with a smile, as he gathered up the stallion's long lead.

"Will do." With a last pat for the bay, the horse climbed up the bank behind Blake. I watched as the pair disappeared from sight.

If only...

But no. Goals were goals and it was crunch time. The culmination of six years of college, with two more to go. Out of the question.

But couldn't a girl have a little fun?

No. Just no.

PRINCE WAS BACK in the corral attached to his trailer when I arrived at Blake's camper. The stallion whuffled softly to me and lipped at the grass I'd found for him. I may be a disaster with men, but I know how to make horses love me. "He'll leave me for you if you keep that up." Blake's eyes glowed down at me from the open door of his camper.

I grinned.

"Come on in and have a drink with me but leave Prince out there. He'd wreck the camper, so he has to stay outside, but you look like you have better manners." He waved me in. "Beer? Juice? Whiskey?"

I thought the juice might be safest in my present state of mind.

The comfortable cab-over camper looked well used, but well cared for. Blake caught me looking it over.

"It's not fancy, but it's gone a lot of miles. We take it camping in the high Sierra and to a lot of endurance rides."

We?

I gulped. Getting ahead of myself again. Of course, a man so vivacious and fun would have a wife. I swallowed the bitter disappointment and accepted the juice with thanks. "High Sierra?"

"Yes, we take the horses and camp up high, near the tree line, and take day rides out from the camper."

I grinned at him beneath my brows. "That's not real camping, in a camper."

He snorted. "Have you ever done it?"

"I've camped for years."

He lifted a brow. "In the high Sierra?"

"Well, no."

"Wait until you try it. You won't think I'm such a tenderfoot, then."

That got me. I had no idea what he meant. And I probably wasn't going to find out. Surely, he was married. Probably to one of those money- grubbers he'd mentioned last time we spoke.

"So, you've finished your meeting?"

"Sure have. I know where I need to be, and when. Stethoscope in hand and secretary assigned. One Janelle Knight."

"Nice girl, Janelle. Known her parents for years. She wants to be a vet."

I shuddered, then grinned. "I'll try not to put her off vet school."

"That tough?"

"Let's just say the course is designed to be passed, but it's tough. Their selection process is strong, so the retention rate is pretty high. So far, out of 134 classmates, we haven't lost any, but we've been lucky enough to gain one from the previous class." I smiled. "Bob had to deal with a pretty steep learning curve when he returned to school after retiring from his naval career—twenty-two *years* after his last college course."

"Most of you weren't even born"—Blake stopped and his

amused look disappeared, then he continued with some hesitation—"when he last studied, then."

What was that about?

I nodded, eyeing Blake sideways.

"Bob's career as a merchant marines engineer was cut short by the Viet Nam draft. Seems the Navy needed marine engineers, so when he was offered a commission in the Navy as an officer, or alternately, to be drafted as an ordinary Army soldier, there wasn't really a choice. The Navy life appealed, so Bob stayed until retirement, but afterwards, he pursued his old dream of becoming a vet of another kind."

"Wow, what dedication."

I smiled. "Yes, he adds so much to our class, every day."

"Let's go or we'll miss dinner." Blake held the door for me as I climbed down the steps.

Gentlemanly.

I didn't see much of that these days. I grinned over my shoulder as I thanked him, then promptly tripped over the trailer brake.

Pull it together. A guy's nice to you and you melt.

I managed to hit the ground with my feet, rather than my head, and stood waiting beside Prince while Blake climbed down—carefully, I noticed.

We headed in the general direction of the cookhouse. Blake stopped at this trailer and that to introduce me to his friends.

The on-duty ambulance rolled slowly to a halt near us, the driver looking around and talking on his radio.

"What's up?" Blake asked someone.

"Faye Waters took her horse out for a ride and her horse came back alone. Not sure what happened, but they found her on the ground, her head against a rock. She had her helmet on, but she was unconscious." He nodded his head at the ambulance. "They've radioed for a chopper and it's on its way. They're finalizing a landing spot now."

The other ambulance attendant hopped out. "Can you all please clear the area? The chopper is on its way," he called out in a loud voice.

We moved to the edge of the clearing and searched the sky for a helicopter. Blake saw it before I could even hear it.

"He's going a pretty good clip." Blake raised an eyebrow at the chopper racing toward us. Suddenly, it was right above us, coming faster than I could have imagined, dropping like a stone into the clearing before us. It was only twenty feet above the ground, too close for comfort. A graying man walked past us, struggling to lead a gray Arabian as it danced sideways, snorting and tugging at its lead. The man glanced around, and then up to see what was frightening his charge. Suddenly, his horse galloped past me, so close I felt the wind from its passing. I turned back to see if the man was okay, but he'd vanished.

Blake dashed off to catch the horse and I ran over to where the man had been. Where had he gone? I peered over the riverbank near where I'd last seen him. There he was. Ten feet down, hunched into a ball on the rocky riverbed, hands and arms cradling his head. His whole body shook.

"Are you all right?" I called out, but he didn't respond. I scrambled down beside him and reached a hand out toward his shoulder.

"No!" Blake's voice rang out from high above me.

I froze, but not before I'd touched the hot skin of the man's shoulder and my world went ballistic. I tried to scream past the fingers digging into my face and covering my mouth, and then a band of flesh-covered steel clamped tight across my throat.

3

Blake leapt off the wall, even as the stranger lunged toward Lena and put her into a chokehold, his fingers reaching for her wildly rolling eyes.

"It's OKAY," Blake yelled at the top of his lungs, jumped down to a patch of sand beside the pair and grabbed for the man's scrabbling free hand. He captured it and held on for grim death, spun the pair around, and twisted the man's arm behind his back.

"No!" The man's voice came out as a sort of a strained croak.

"Let go of the girl, you're both safe," said Blake in the calmest, most level voice he could muster. The man must be mostly deaf.

Lena's captor took one deep breath and then another, then his grip on Lena seemed to loosen.

"Lena, don't move." Blake whispered. "Just stay still."

The girl shook, but she remained frozen, her back to the two men. The only movement was the chopper's vibration of the air, and of the very ground.

"I'm back," the stranger said, his voice cracking and rusty.

He released Lena and she stood like a rock, frozen in place.

"You're a returned serviceman?" Blake's loud question was more of a statement, and the man gave a faint nod. "Okay, I'm letting go now. Do you want to talk about it?"

He shook his head and glanced up from the ground toward Lena. "I'm sorry, ma'am." His gravelly voice was barely audible.

She turned to the man and reached out her hand. "Nothing to forgive," she said, as tears filled her eyes. "Was it the chopper?"

He flinched, then squared his shoulders. "I'm okay now."

Blake placed his hand firmly on the man's shoulder. "Can I do anything for—"

"MARK!" A blonde woman, tears streaming down her red, sweaty face, jumped down the embankment in two hops. Pulling him into her arms, she rocked him like a baby. "Are you all right?" She fairly shouted into his ear.

He nodded, slowly. "I thought it was a Snake," he barely got out.

"I saw the chopper show up and got here as fast as I could," she puffed. "Lord knows what they think back at the registration desk, but I don't care. I had to find you."

"These nice people," Mark grated, "helped me. I'm afraid I scared the young lady when she surprised me—"

"No harm done," Lena barked and turned to the woman. "Anything we can do to help?" she continued, in a softer voice. "Shall I go get your horse?"

"Nothing anyone can do," the woman growled softly, "except be there for him. It's the choppers. The horse will be back at the trailer with his buddy by now. He knows the score—and he's less scared of choppers than Mark is."

Blake assessed the man's age—about the same as his own. "Was he in Nam?"

The blonde nodded and kept rocking.

"I was there, too. I understand. If you both feel like it, come find us later. We'll be at the white trailer with the attached corral and the bay stallion. You're both welcome."

The sound of the chopper's rotors changed. The woman gulped and gripped Mark even more tightly.

"Thank you for being there for him." She took a deep breath and backed away from her man, just far enough to lock eyes with him. "You're okay. Hold on to me, that chopper's heading out now. The ambulance crew already had Faye strapped into the stretcher, so they'll just head straight out." She gripped him to her with what looked like all her strength as the chopper blades whipped the air and dirt around them into a gritty cloud, then it was gone, the intense noise fading into the trees like it'd never been.

Mark filled his lungs and turned his face to Lena and Blake, though he never let go of his woman. "We'll see you tonight," he said, and let the blonde lead him away.

Lena stared at Blake after they'd gone, her pupils so wide that her green eyes looked black.

"You okay?" Blake said, his voice sounding rough to his ears. He wanted to reach out to her but held back.

"I've never experienced anything like…" Her voice trailed off.

"And it's a blessing you've never had to," Blake cut in, letting himself reach for her hand. She gripped it with surprising strength.

"Will you tell me about—"

"No." It came out more brusquely than he'd meant, and she inhaled sharply, glancing up from the hand he still held.

"I'm—"

"No. I didn't mean it that way." He filled his lungs and slowly let the air drain away. "The fact you've never been exposed to anything like that, as I said, is a blessing, and please god you never will. It marks you for life. You're never the same again,"—he glanced at the retreating backs of the blonde and Mark—"mentally or physically."

"Poor man," she murmured. Her tears flowed freely now. With a sort of grim admiration, he watched the girl who'd held up under pressure yet still had the depth of feeling to crumple when the threat was past.

If only...

He shook himself.

No. She has too much life to live yet.

But... he hesitated... she needed comfort, anyway. "Come here." Blake pulled her into his arms for a hug but released her as she stiffened. "Let's go, eh?" He found an easy way up the bank and climbed up, then put a hand down to her. "Let's find some supper before the rest of them eat it all."

His thoughts jumbled as they walked toward the sounds of clanging pots and clinking silverware. She was fun, bright—and just starting out. He sighed as his heart squeezed tight in his chest. And she was young. Probably too young for him. He glanced down at the top of her shining brunette head. It would just end up like last time... in tears. She was far too pretty for it to be otherwise.

Nice thought, Sagan.

He shook his head to clear it and walked on, packing more stuffing around his heart in the hope that would keep it safe.

I LEANED FORWARD, closer to the light of Blake's campfire later that evening to make sure my marshmallow was browning and not turning into a flaming torch.

"Haven't had marshmallows in years." Blake's satisfied murmur warmed me. "Thanks for bringing them. Great idea."

"Hello," came a gravelly voice from the edge of the firelight.

"Hey, you two, pull up a stump," Blake said, as Mark and his blonde ladyfriend walked into the light of the campfire.

"How's your horse?" I shouted, with as much warmth as I could muster. "He didn't find any trouble running around camp by himself, did he?"

"No," Mark said, looking down at the ground with a little smile, "and I'd like to introduce you to Wendy. I wasn't much of myself earlier today."

We both greeted Wendy, talking until Mark spoke again.

"I wanted to thank you both. They really throw me, the choppers. Doesn't matter what kind—they all feel like Snakes to me." He fell silent and Wendy took his hand, then moved her log seat closer.

"Do you want to talk about it?" Blake's voice was gentle.

Mark nodded, but didn't speak for long moments.

"Would anyone like something to drink?" I looked around the circle. "I've brought homemade chocci-chip cookies, too."

"We brought our drinks, but thanks, I'd love a cookie," Wendy said, as a smile broke out on Mark's face.

"Yes, thanks," Mark said, as I leapt to my feet for the container of munchies.

Mark took a deep breath and let it out slowly. "You sure you don't mind my talking about it?" He looked at Blake, who smiled and reached out a hand to pat him on the shoulder, then sat back down beside me.

"I fought in the jungle in Nam... for too long." Mark winced and went on after a few moments. "Lucky to have survived. The Vietcong were like wraiths, appearing where there'd been no one a moment before. That was terrifying enough, but it was the choppers that got to me. There really weren't frontlines defining 'us' versus 'them' most of the time, so our fighters couldn't just go in and bomb everything. They had to fly in low—just over the treetops or the elephant grass —in their little Loaches to see exactly who it was on the ground." He stopped and took a sip of his bottle of beer. After another deep breath, he went on. "When the pilots of the Loaches saw a target, or some men they wanted to bomb, they'd drop a smoke flare and clear out. Within seconds, a Cobra,"—he glanced up at Blake—"we called 'em Snakes, would fly over and rocket the crap out of the area." His voice quavered to a halt and he shook his head.

"You don't have to go on," Wendy murmured.

"Yes, I do," he hissed, then squeezed her hand and kissed it. "I want to get over this… not talking about it hasn't worked either, but thank you, anyway."

Wendy swallowed hard. Her knuckles over her man's fist glowed white in the firelight as Mark continued.

"A Loach went right past me and suddenly the air was full of smoke," he mumbled. "I knew what was coming, but I couldn't get away fast enough." He fell silent again. "The bomb hit—too close, *way* too close. I got burned pretty badly. Then my time came up for the R & R flight the airlines organized—took me and a bunch of the other boys to Australia. When my time was over, back I went." He swallowed hard and took another sip.

"How long were you there?" I finally asked into the gap in the talk.

"When most of the troops left in the '73 withdrawal, I stayed behind as security for the embassy. How long? Seemed like forever, but it didn't much matter." He fell silent, and it stretched out to minutes. "Didn't have any family to go home to," he said, with abrupt finality.

No one moved a muscle until he spoke again.

"Just before the North Vietnamese took over a couple years later, I had a girlfriend who worked for Pan Am. Seems Pan Am had promised they'd get all of their people out and she tried to get me onto a special volunteer mercy mission they flew—after the airports were already shut down—but I was a guard for the ambassador at the US Embassy and the ambassador'd been good to me…" Mark stopped again and stared into the fire. "I don't think I'll ever hear 'White Christmas' again without tearing up.

"When the NVA were nearly at the gates of the Presidential Palace, we pulled out for good. Thousands of Americans and South Vietnamese wanted to get out before the North Vietnamese took over—they were afraid of being executed or sent to one of the famous NVA 'reeducation camps'. The airstrips were all destroyed, so a mass evacuation by plane was out. Air America and the Marines flew all night through thunderstorms and evacuated seven thousand people by *chopper*. I was guarding the embassy building that night, quaking in my boots at the sound of the choppers flying in and out. They landed on whatever roofs would hold them and hovered over the others, loading up all the refugees they could carry. Ambassador Martin was a good man. Yep, a good man." He nodded vehemently. "A Marine in a chopper landed on the embassy roof helicopter pad and asked for him, but instead of coming up himself, the ambassador sent up Vietnamese and other non-U.S. evacuees, and the Marine guards had to load *them* into the chopper and fly them out to the USS Blue Ridge. Not once, but again and again. Every time they landed, the ambassador kept sending his staff and other Vietnamese. He knew the flight he left on would be the last one out, so he stayed in the building.

"Around five in the morning, when the same pilot landed for the umpteenth time, he called the embassy sergeant over while the guards were loading his chopper with refugees again. He told the sergeant the chopper wasn't leaving until the ambassador was aboard." Mark looked up at all of us. " 'Get these refugees off and bring Ambassador Martin either freely or under arrest' the pilot said. I remember it like it was yesterday, and he added 'the president sends', which probably wasn't true, but it worked.

"So how'd you get out, Mark?" Wendy said, gripping his arm.

"The ambassador took me with him, but if he hadn't grabbed my jacket and held on, I wouldn't have gotten anywhere within 100 yards of that chopper. I heard the pilot saying he'd been flying for over eighteen hours straight—including fourteen trips to the embassy." A faint smile played upon his lips. "Later that day, I took great pleasure in helping everyone push choppers off the USS Blue Ridge into the sea."

"Pushing choppers off?" Wendy stared.

Mark shrugged. "With all the refugees on board, there wasn't enough space for more choppers to land."

He leaned back and shared a long look with Wendy, then turned back to Blake and me. "So you see why I don't do helicopters. I lived, but anytime I hear a chopper, or see one…" He gave a sigh so massive I could almost see the tension flow out of him. "When I have some warning, I can hold on, but otherwise… as you've seen, I can't."

I let out the breath I didn't know I'd been holding and reached for the hand Wendy wasn't already gripping for dear life and squeezed.

Mark gave us the hint of a smile. "Thanks for listening, all… maybe… this will help."

"You're alive, man." Blake reached out to place a hand, almost in benediction, upon Mark's shoulder.

Mark looked around our circle in the firelight and lifted his bottle. "I give thanks for that. Most of those from my units aren't. Don't know how or why I've been spared, but sometimes I wonder. Lots of better men than me died."

"Who's to say?" Blake said softly. "All you can do is live your life well."

"The horses have been good for me—they make up for a

lot." Mark looked sideways at Wendy, who flushed when he said, "and so do you."

"Don't I know that." Blake's eyes in the flames' flickering light were haunted for a moment, then the look was gone.

What was that about?

They sat in silence for a few minutes, only the sound of crackling flames consuming wood, the stamp of a random hoof against the ground, and the steady rhythmic chomp of horses chewing their supper.

"We'd best get off to bed, folks," Mark said with a smile. "Not as young as I used to be. Thank you again for the hospitality and the friendship."

"Anytime. We'll be seeing you tomorrow," Blake said, standing to see them off. I waved and sat back down.

"You okay?" I murmured, when he'd sat back down.

Blake didn't answer for a moment. "Yep. Fine." Abruptly.

I swallowed hard. He didn't sound it, but who was I to pry where it wasn't wanted?

He looked up at me and smiled, but it was more of a grimace. "Best I head for bed too, much as I'd like to stay up and talk. Rain check for tomorrow? Four a.m. feeding for Prince will come early."

"It sure will." I twisted the tail of my shirt in one hand. "Thank you for the campfire and the talk, Blake. I enjoyed it."

"Not the most pleasant of topics, but…" Blake's gaze was lost to the fire. "It's all fine." He tightened his jaw and stood.

"Don't get up, enjoy your fire." A niggle of discomfort at his unease ran up my spine and I shivered.

"Hard to walk you back to your tent if I don't." His eyes shone in the light of the lantern and his luminous smile lit up the night brighter than any artificial lantern.

"You don't have to do that," I protested.

Lowered brows and a look of confusion. "Of course, I do. My mother raised a gentleman and I don't intend to change."

I smiled. This was a first. "Thank you then, kind sir." I gave him a half bow and preceded him from the camp.

"Thanks for listening tonight..." Blake hesitated, then went on. "I'm sure it made a difference to Mark. It did to me." He took my hand and squeezed it, then with a whispered "goodnight," he left me.

Blake had looked so sad tonight. My heart squeezed in my chest just thinking of it. His campsite was within view of the open door of my tent, and I couldn't help watching as he returned to his temporary home. Blake's outline, highlighted by the campfire light, disappeared into his camper for only a minute, then it returned to stand alongside his horse for long minutes, his arms wrapped around the bay's neck. It was still there when I let the tent flap drop, leaving him to his thoughts. I hoped he'd get some rest—he looked like he needed it, and he had fifty miles to ride tomorrow. I was thankful he had Prince.

4

"Lena," said the head ride veterinarian, Seth Latimer, the next morning, "I know you're only here to do P & Rs, but can you please keep an eye out for metabolic problems?"

"Sure can, no problem." I nodded.

"Specifically, we'll be watching for dehydration, capillary refill time, and decreased gut sounds," Dr. Latimer said, "and we've only got two vets here today, so we're a little understaffed. With your Large Animal ICU experience, you're a godsend."

I smiled, right down to my heart. With two more years of vet school left, my dream of actually becoming a veterinarian still seemed a long way away, but his comment helped me believe it was all real and *would* actually happen. It had taken such a very long time.

Finally.

"Here's your radio," he said. "If you need me, I'm on number one and Dr. Grant is Vet Two. You're Vet Three. You have my permission to hold and check any horse that concerns you. Try to contact me with any concerns, but if you can't find me, pull in Dr. Grant. This race is running under AERC rules, so the vets are the control judges and we, or I, anyway, have the last word.

"Sounds good. Do you expect trouble?"

"With this heat,"—he wiped his brow, already sweating in the early light—"we're bound to have problems if the riders get too competitive and don't take care of their horses."

My jaw clenched. In a human sport, people could make their own decisions, but riders could easily push an animal beyond its fitness level or capabilities. That's why vets are in charge here. To keep the riders from pushing their horses, or to keep the keener horses from killing themselves during the fifty miles of the race. It wasn't a hundred-miler, but fifty miles wasn't exactly a walk in the park. The horses would need to be well-conditioned to have a chance of staying well.

"Now you know the weather conditions, what will the P & R criteria be today?" I asked.

"I'll go over that in,"—he glanced at his watch—"ten minutes at the pre-ride talk, but their pulses have to be down to 60 after a trot out within half an hour of coming into a vet check, and of course, they have to be metabolically stable and sound at a trot." He turned toward his truck, then spun back. "You have a thermometer? Everyone remembers stethoscopes, but the thermometers often get left at home."

"Always." I patted the EMT belt pouch at my side.

"Then let's head over to the meeting. It's nearly time."

The meeting passed uneventfully, then the riders headed back to their trailers for their final preparations. As we left in Dr. Latimer's truck for the first vet check, horses and riders were already assembling near the starting line.

The big Ford with a vet pack on the back bounced over the ruts and bumps of what passed for a road, jarring bones at every pothole, on the way to vet check number one.

"Would've been a smoother ride"—I glanced at him—"on a horse."

"Yeah, well, you're right, but we might need some of the gear in back. Hopefully not, but... you never know your luck. The meds might look like a milkshake, though."

"Activated." I grinned.

"So, have you got a job lined up for after graduation?"

I shook my head. "Haven't started looking yet, but I had a great preceptorship in the Santa Ynez Valley in a big surgical practice. They cut a lot of colic surgeries and did plenty of orthopedic and stud work."

"Which did you prefer?"

"I enjoyed the surgery and the stud work, but I'm leaning toward a practice where I can work with individual owners and their horses—horses they'd like to keep going for many years."

"Racetrack and stud work don't appeal to you? It's a much more glamorous life." He raised a brow at me.

"I'll do them if I must,"—I shook my head—"but I prefer pleasure and competition horses on a smaller scale—glamour doesn't do it for this small-town girl, I guess."

"I like the way you think, Lena. Private owners need good vets too. Don't ever let anyone tell you you'd be wasted on them." He smiled at me as he parked the truck, then pointed out the P & R area. "Sarah will get you set up. First horses should be in"—he glanced at his watch again—"right about now."

Within five minutes, a big rangy bay mare with a dark-haired woman aboard trotted in, first through the gate.

The timer consulted his stopwatch, then wrote her number and time down on his clipboard and on her rider card, then she continued on to her crew who'd set up a temporary camp near us.

The man quickly sponged the horse while the other crew member, a teenaged boy, swapped a full water bottle for the rider's empty one and checked the bay's legs, then the woman's saddle and bridle.

"Going well?" the boy asked.

"She's flying. Left the others way behind." The rider glanced up to see the second horse come past the timer, then glanced at the stopwatch she wore around her neck. "Check her heart rate, please, love?" she asked the man as the boy handed her a paper-wrapped packet and she stuffed it into the neckline of her shirt. "Thanks darling, I'll eat it on the trail."

The man produced a stethoscope from around his neck and slid its head behind the mare's left elbow while the woman stroked the horse's head and neck. His lips moved as he multiplied the rate. "She's good to go. Head on over to P & R."

My brows raised. She must be fit if she was already ready to go through.

"Well done, crew. We're off." The rider smiled at her team. "P & R, please?" she called, as she walked the horse toward us.

"Over here, thanks," I said. When she reached us, she handed her card to my secretary, Kim. "She's recovered quickly." I closed my eyes to listen to the mare's heart.

The rider laughed. "It's funny to see everyone close their eyes to listen to a heart rate."

"Fifty-four," I said, to Kim, and grinned at the dark-haired woman. "But we all do it—it helps me focus on the quality of the sound, but it *is* funny, you're right."

While I counted her respiratory rate, I pulled a bit of skin out and watched it retract over the point of her shoulder to check for dehydration, then lifted her lip to press a finger against the mare's gums for her capillary refill time. "How's she going out there?" I asked the rider, who couldn't be more than a hundred pounds soaking wet. This big mare wouldn't even notice her weight.

"54/16," I said to my secretary. She jotted it down and

handed the card back to the rider. "She's looking great, and you're good to go. Have a nice ride."

With a cheery smile and a wave of thanks, the girl walked the horse away a few steps, then clucked her tongue. The mare pricked up her ears and set off at a lope from a standstill as the woman vaulted on and they disappeared at a canter.

"She's serious about this, isn't she? What a team," I said to Kim as I glanced at her crew. They'd already packed up and were halfway back to their truck.

"They're going for AERC Top Ten Award for the year. It's certainly not out of their reach."

I shook my head with a smile. "Lovely to see that sort of care for a horse."

"It's their trademark," Kim said.

"Time to get busy," I said as more horses came through the gate.

"P & R," called the second-place rider, and our teammates headed to take care of him.

It wasn't long before the horses were coming through hard and fast. There was no time for idle chit-chat, but having ridden plenty of these races, I knew how much riders appreciate a smile and a well-wishing upon their exit. The day progressed like that—quiet periods of joking around with the P & R teams, then rushing to get everyone checked.

"Lena, let's go on to the next check," called Dr. Latimer, and we headed for his truck. "How have the horses been?"

"So far," I said, "they're looking great."

Doc Latimer grinned, probably at my rampant enthusiasm. "What did you think of that first horse?"

"She's a stunner, and what a crew!"

A slow smile. "They're in my practice. A better crew you won't find. Her son has a very good six-year-old he's bringing on. He'll be ready to compete next year... and he'll give

Karen, his mom, a run for her money. Best thing is, Karen'll love it."

"Does his dad ride? I take it that's him?"

"Jake doesn't ride, but he loves to crew. He can't wait to crew for them both… but as he tells them all the time, they'll have to both be top notch or he can't be there for them both."

"He's got a point," I said, with a wry grin.

"Nice family. They take fantastic care of their horses. The best. They deserve to win races… and they do win."

IT WAS all on at the next vet check. Horses came and went as fast as we could check them and sign them off.

Blake and Prince stayed within the top ten throughout the morning. At the first check, our group checked them and at the next, one of the other teams had the chance to listen to his heart and lungs, but everyone agreed, Prince's recovery times were astonishing.

"And I have to admit," I said to the others, after Prince trotted out the gate, "I thought he was too out of condition to race. I was *so* wrong." I chuckled.

"Those Polish Arabs are the best," said Vanessa, a girl on my P & R team.

"P & R?" another rider called.

I could only nod as we hurried over to the next horse.

Mark and his gray Arabian were about the thirtieth team to come through the second check. Mark looked so ecstatic, I could hardly reconcile him with the distraught man beside the campfire last night.

"How's your horse going?" I asked him.

"Doing great, and so am I. Thanks for last night, Lena, and please give my best to Blake, too, from both of us."

"Any time. Hope to catch up with you later," I said as I placed the stethoscope over his horse's heart.

I pulled the stethoscope out of my ears and told the secretary the horse's heart rate.

"Sorry, but we have to head out as soon as we're finished, so we probably won't see you, but let's get together sometime?" Mark said, as he led his gray away. "Thanks again," he called, beaming around at the world.

We were about to pack up and head for the third vet check when Jared, one of the other P & R team members, tapped me on the shoulder.

"Lena," he said, as I looked up, "number 79 is due to come back to be checked and hasn't shown. Should I send someone to look for them?"

"Yes, thanks." I turned back to the horse I'd just clamped a stethoscope on. "60/18," I reported. Kim noted it down as I thanked the rider while checking the skin turgor and refill, then wished her well with a wave.

"I found number 79," Jared said, beside my ear. "I think you need to check him. He doesn't look so good and his rider says his pulse isn't coming down."

"Okay, Jared. Can you take over here please?" I waved goodbye to him and Kim, throwing back over my shoulder, "there aren't any vets at this check anymore, are there?"

Jared shook his head with a grimace. "Doc Latimer had to go on, but he said to find you if there were any horses needing to be checked."

"I'll go see the horse. Call if you need me." I pulled out my radio. "Vet Three to Vet One, come in Vet One."

"Vet One," Dr. Latimer's voice crackled over the speaker. "What've you got?"

I told him.

"Okay, let me know. I'm ten minutes away, out."

"Out."

The bay Morgan gelding drooped, his head hanging low, and he didn't even glance up as I approached. His eyes were dull and incurious, as if he didn't care what was happening around him.

I introduced myself to the middle-aged female rider. "How has he been going?"

"He was fine until an hour ago, then he seemed tired all of a sudden."

"Are you his rider?"

"Yes." Shortly.

"Has he done this before? In your training rides?"

"Ummm… haven't had much time to trail him lately," she said, her eyes everywhere but my face.

I gulped and tried to unclench my jaws. Unfit and still racing, on a 104-degree day? I forced myself to stay calm.

"Is he drinking? Eating?" I looked around the area to see an untouched hay net and no water bucket in sight.

She stared at me. "What is this, *20 Questions?*"

"I'm trying to ascertain the condition of your horse"—I placed the stethoscope on the horse's chest and shut my eyes —"and anything you can tell me would help."

"You're a vet?"

"Vet student."

"Get away from my horse," she squeaked.

I blinked and stepped back. "Dr. Latimer asked me to evaluate your horse and let him know what I find. He's at the next vet check, ten minutes away."

She eyed me sideways. "Okay, check him. He didn't want any water at the last stop, so my crew didn't get him any this time."

I tried not to shriek as I moved back to the horse's girth. His heart rate was way too high, 72 beats per minute. Fast and thready.

"He can't be dehydrated," she snapped. "He stopped sweating miles back."

My heart stopped in its tracks. It didn't get much worse. I tented the skin over the horse's shoulder and the skin took several seconds to slide back. I swallowed hard. Moving my stethoscope to his flank, I listened in vain for gut sounds, but the regular, progressive gurgling sounds of borborygmus were absent and his capillary refill time was three seconds. I'd seen better CRTs in a nearly-dead horse. This one was in trouble. I slid the thermometer into his backside and waited while I stroked his dull coat with my other hand. When I pulled it out, I blinked. 39 degrees. Off scale.

"He's not looking so good," I said to the woman. "I'm going to radio Dr. Latimer. Can you see if he'll drink some electrolyte water, please? How much electrolyte water has he had today?"

No answer.

"Yesterday?" I was close to pleading now. "Salt block?"

"I don't use any of those things. Look, what's the matter with the lazy sod?"

"I'll let the vet speak with you about this, if you don't mind," I said, trying not to growl at her. Ignorance was no excuse in this game, and I didn't trust myself to not deck her for abusing and neglecting this horse.

"Vet Three to Vet One, come in," I barked as I walked away. I had to get far, far away from the rider.

"Vet One here. How's the horse?"

"Any worse and he'd be dead," I muttered as soon as I was out of hearing range of the rider. "Heart rate 72, depressed, dehydrated, no gut sounds, not eating or drinking at last check, so didn't offer it at this one. I've sent a girl for water, but his eyes are glazed and he's past caring. His temp's 39 degrees." We need you back here, Doc. You have fluids?"

"Yes. On my way," he said. A truck door slammed and an engine revved as he signed off.

"Dr. Latimer's on his way," I said to the woman and spun to borrow a bucket and sponge. This horse needed a cooldown.

So did I.

5

"My professional opinion?" Dr. Latimer's voice, as he spoke with the irate owner of the exhausted horse, was so soft as to be barely audible, but the thinly-veiled fury was unmistakable.

"Yes, what's the matter with my horse?"

"I'm glad you asked. Plain and simple, he's been pushed past his fitness level and you're in very real danger of losing him, especially if we don't pull off some heroics here. Do we have your permission to begin?"

The rider of horse number 79 threw up her arms and stalked away. "Do what you need to," she threw over her shoulder. "I'm going to take a nap. It's been a long day."

The young teenager crewing for her stood looking at the retreating woman's back, tears in her eyes, then she ran to the bay and wrapped her arms around his neck, sobbing as if her heart would break.

Dr. Latimer turned to me. "You go see what you can do for the girl, I'll get the truck."

I nodded and approached the pair. "We'll do whatever we can for him. What is his name, and yours?" I said softly.

"Sara," she said, between sobs, "and Sabado." She reached for the bucket to offer him water again. He lipped at it listlessly, but didn't drink, and just leaned his head against hers.

"Is that your mother?"

"My *step*mother," she spat from between gritted teeth, then stepped back to slip the girth and pull his saddle off. She grabbed the towel tucked into the back pocket of her jeans and began to rub him down.

"Does she do much endurance with her horse?"

"Sabado is *my* horse," she growled, reaching for the halter to replace Sabado's bridle. "Tracey"—she thrust her chin in the direction of their camper—"heard about this ride and wanted to enter, so she did. My dad is away, and she wouldn't tell me his new phone number." Sara stood still, her eyes staring into the distance as she spoke. "This horse is my everything. He's only fit for the show ring and trail rides with an empathetic rider. My mother and I broke him in together. I was the first to ride him. The *only* one to ride him until Tracey came along—and Dad won't do a thing about it. I begged her not to take him in this race, but you see how she is." Her face was set.

Dr. Latimer backed his vet truck right up to them and the horse didn't even lift his head.

"Sara, do you have some clean water in a clean bucket?" I asked her, and she stirred.

"My first aid kit has a new garbage bag to line a bucket, *and* electrolytes."

"Great," I smiled at her, "Can you get it right away?"

With a kiss on her horse's forehead, she bolted.

"If you get me a cutthroat razor and some scrub, I'll prep him for a catheter—two, probably, 14 gauge?"

His brows shot up, then his grimace cracked into a smile. "I forgot you're an ICU tech. Fantastic. Go for it—I'll get the fluids set up." He handed me the scrub supplies and set up a folding table beside me.

I told him what Sara had said.

"The lying..." He clamped his mouth shut in a hard line as he placed catheters and a T-port onto the table top.

"Some suture and an 18 gauge needle is all I'll need," I said as he prepared to open a surgical pack.

"No needle holders?"

I shook my head and glanced up at the sound of running feet. "Oh, Sara, do you have some braid bands?"

"Sure thing," she said with a tortured look at her horse and spun away again.

I quickly scrubbed and shaved over Sabado's jugulars on both sides, the hair slicing cleanly away under the straight-edged razor.

"I've got them." Sara held out the bag of small black rubber bands.

"Can you make some long braids, one down each side, just behind his bridle path?"

She looked askance at me, but she did as I'd asked and tied the ends off with her bands while I prepped the catheter sites.

"Can you get some tape from Dr. Latimer?"

She was back in a moment and I told her how to make loops from the main braids to hold the IV lines. As she completed that task, I blocked the catheter areas and four points surrounding them with a fine needle and local anesthetic.

"Poor Sabado." Sara bit her lip. "He never even moved when you stuck him."

I bit my lip, then returned my focus to my table. I gloved up and soon the first catheter slid into place.

"I have your fluids ready, 'Doc'." He nodded up at the fluid bags tied high on the side of Sara's horse trailer.

I smiled. "Thanks. Some suture please, and that needle?" I

screwed the T-port snugly to the catheter and held it against the horse's neck, then glanced up to see Dr. Latimer watching closely, holding up a suture cartridge and the needle. With a pair of forceps, he drew some suture out till I nodded, cut it, and handed it over. Looping the material in one gloved hand, I asked him to open the needle case. I grabbed the needle hub, while he held on to the cap, and I slid it into the already-blocked skin beneath the T-port.

"Ah, that's how you do it. I've always used needle holders and a cutting needle."

"Easier this way, and they stay in better. The sutures don't cut through the skin so easily. We do them like this in ICU."

"Very tidy." Dr. Latimer nodded his approval then threaded one of the IV lines through Sabado's top halter ring, looped it twice through one mane loop, and attached it to the T-port. "I pulled some blood while you were busy here, so we have a baseline, anyway. I have a microhematocrit in the truck, so we can at least check his PCV."

Reaching up, he turned the drip set to full and it flowed like a little river, delivering life-giving fluid to the dehydrated horse.

"Go ahead and run the bloods while I put the second line in, if you want," I said.

"I can help with the IV line," Sara said, from my elbow. "I watched Dr. Latimer do it."

"Sure." I smiled down at her face, all big eyes and worry lines. "I'd love the help."

"And just for the record," Sara said, "he wasn't well at the last stop and didn't want to drink, so she wouldn't *let* me give him any this time—said she'd teach him… and now she's probably *killed* him." She finished on a wail, then collected herself.

My heart ached for the girl. "When is your father back home?"

"He should be home tomorrow," she whispered. "I miss him so much. He'll be heartbroken. Sabado's mother was Mom's pride and joy."

I didn't dare ask any more about either of them. The girl was holding together, but by her shaking hands and quivering lip, it was a near thing.

By the time we ran fifteen liters into Sabado, he started to perk up and his gut sounds returned. Sluggish, but returned, and his temperature had dropped. When his PCV fell to something near normal range, we slowed the fluids. After twenty liters, he ate the handful of grass Sara picked for him and looked around for more.

Dr. Grant radioed to say Blake and Prince came across the finish line first, followed closely by the second to fifth-placed horses. All else was well.

My heart leapt at the news.

"Nice horse, that Prince," Dr. Latimer's face relaxed into a grin. "Lives for him, does Blake."

"He seems an awfully nice man." I smiled inwardly. "We met yesterday. Do you do his regular vet work?"

"Sure do, though he's nearly an hour away from me. No other equine vets up that way." He looked sideways at me but didn't say more.

We capped his T-ports and flushed them, then watched Sara lead him away to pick at any grass they could find.

"He's still not as alert as I'd like to see," Dr. Latimer said, "but he's alive."

I nodded.

"One of us has to stay here and run Sabado more fluids, at least until he starts to urinate again"—he hesitated—"and I don't want you subjected to that woman on your own." His lips tightened as he glanced toward the silent camper. "It's a blessing Sabado happened to crash here, rather than somewhere inaccessible."

"He's a lot brighter," Sara said, as she led the horse up to them, "and he's eating... do you... do you think he'll be all right?" The pleading in her voice made me want to cry.

"Honestly, Sara, he's not out of the woods yet, but when he's fully hydrated, I'll give him some anti-inflammatories to try to ward off any potential complications, but he *is* looking a lot better."

"Potential complications"—the girl swallowed hard —"like.... like colic and... laminitis?" This last was said in a whisper.

Dr. Latimer's eyes narrowed at her and his jaw clenched. After a deep breath, he spoke. "Yes, Sara. You sound like you've seen this before?"

"Yes." Flat. Final. She tied Sabado back to the trailer. "You're giving him more fluids now?"

"Yes... Sara, I've got him here, why don't you go with Lena to the finish line for awhile?"

She looked at him with horror. "Leave Sabado?"

"I'll be with him... I want to speak with your stepmom alone."

"Oh." She shivered. "Okay, then." With another hug around Sabado's neck, she walked to the front of their truck and grabbed a jacket. I got mine and put it on as we walked. With the evening's approach, the temperature was dropping rapidly.

"Lena!"

I turned to see Blake leading Prince toward me, his head and back swinging. Beside me, Sara sighed.

"What?" I asked her.

"What a beautiful horse." She smiled.

"He is."

"He's just finished the fifty miles?" She stared at Prince as he neared them.

"He's just *won* it."

Sara blinked. "But he looks so... so *well*." She swallowed hard and tears filled her eyes.

"Yes, he's fit for it, and a stallion to boot," I said. "Doc's taking care of your boy. It's all we can do right now."

She took a deep breath and looked at Prince. "He's lovely and looks full of life."

"Congratulations, Blake," I said, and wrapped my arms around Prince's neck. "And to you, Prince." Lifting my head, I met Blake's gaze squarely. "And I have to give it to you, you're right. He looks like he's been for a trot down the road to the store and back. No different from the way he looked yesterday." My grin was so wide I thought my face would split.

His eyes glowed at me for a moment before he turned to Sara. I introduced them while I rubbed Prince's forehead, or rather, he rubbed his forehead on me. I finished with, "I normally wouldn't let a horse rub on me like this, but he's earned it today."

"He sure has," Blake said, then turned back to the girl. "Sara, your dad's first name isn't Kent, is it?"

She narrowed her brows at him. "Yes, why?"

"I used to fly with him. How's he going, and your mom? Haven't seen you since you were just a little tyke."

"Dad's away, but mom's... mom's...."

"Blake," I stared hard at him, "Sara's horse was in the race, ridden by her *step*mother."

He took the hint. "How did the horse do?"

A stony silence met him.

"Dr. Latimer's been treating him. Heat exhaustion, dehydration..." I fell silent.

"Lena has been helping a lot," Sara said proudly, with an ineffective swipe at the tears in her eyes and I smiled at her.

"Where *is* the good doc?"

"He's still with Sara's horse," I murmured. "And hopefully talking some sense into Tracey."

"Tracey..." Blake froze.

"She was Tracey Brownlea."

Blake let out his breath and looked at Sara. "So, is your horse going to be okay? Which horse is it?"

"If you remember my mom, it's the son of her mare. Sabado."

Blake smiled at her. "He was a beautiful and trusting foal. But why did you let Tracey..."

"Blake, don't you need to get ready to go back for Best Condition judging? They'll be starting"—I glanced at my watch—"soon," I said pointedly, with a sideways look at Sara, who looked like she wanted the ground to open up and swallow her.

His brow lowered as he flicked a glance my way, and then toward the girl. "Yes, do you two want to come?"

Sara's hopeful gaze fastened on him and she glanced at Prince. "Do you have a towel? He needs a tidy-up first."

"We'll get one when we go past the truck. It seems"—he smiled at me—"we have a team member who knows how to pretty up a horse."

After they arrived back at the trailer, Blake sent Sara for a small bucket of clean water.

"But we have a tank on board," I said, after the girl had trotted off with her bucket.

He glanced at Sara's retreating back. "Tracey, her stepmother, is one of those money-grubbing ones I mentioned. I wondered why she finally got the message I didn't want her hanging around. She found herself another pilot."

"Poor man, and poor Sara... and Sabado," was all I could say.

"And so," I said to Raywyn with a grin, which of course she couldn't see beneath my mask while I prepped a dog for surgery on the following Tuesday, "not only did Prince win the race, but he also won Best Condition."

"So, tell me about Blake," Ray said, with a sly sideways look, and handed me another disinfectant-soaked gauze with her gleaming steel forceps.

"What about him?" I hedged.

"I can't see your lips, but your eyes are glowing." She watched my motions as I swabbed the dog's abdomen from my planned incision line in a circular outward motion and made a little correction.

"Is this right?" I asked.

"Yes, better."

"A good vet tech is worth more than a hundred textbooks in true learning value."

"Good to know I'm appreciated but stop changing the subject."

I snorted behind the blue fabric.

"So, when will you see him again?" Ray was relentless.

This should stop her.

"Next weekend."

She blinked. "Truly? Where?"

"At his ranch." Smug.

"But where?"

"Elk Valley Springs, Tehachapi."

"But that's over two hours away!"

"Just seeing his *horse* is worth it—Blake's a bonus." I giggled. It'd been a long time since I'd felt so good.

"It's wonderful to see you happy"—her brows lowered —"but are you sure you know what you're doing, I mean, you just met the guy, and… you're going to his place for the weekend? What do you really know about him? He could…" Ray gulped "Be a—"

"It'll be okay, he's an old-fashioned gentleman," I interrupted.

The little voice inside my head said it too…

Yeah, you don't even know the guy.

"I'll be fine. I always am."

"Famous last words." Ray cocked a brow at me. "Ready to start this surgery? I'll get Dr. Franco and he can observe you."

"Thanks." I smiled at her. Good friends weren't easy to come by and Ray was one in a million. But was Ray right? What could life be like with a gentleman like Blake? Surely, I'd not done anything to deserve that kind of care and attention.

But maybe, just maybe…

6

Somehow, the week flew by, a million dogs and cats, plus the occasional bird and reptile. Before I knew it, it was Friday. I threw the last bag, full of riding clothes, helmet, and boots, onto the back seat and waved goodbye to Ray.

With Gordon Lightfoot and me blasting out songs from *Gord's Gold* on the truck stereo, windows all the way down, the tension of the week just slid away. As much as I love cats and dogs, I could never be a small animal vet. Horses are it for me. Always have been and probably always will.

My excitement grew as I climbed from the valley floor into the Tehachapi Mountains, heading away to play with horses and get to know a new friend. Despite whatever I seemed to be thinking, that's all it could be... for now.

I turned onto Elk Valley Springs Road and blinked. Blake told me there was a gateway... but a gated *community*? I stopped before the big metal sliding gate beside a guardhouse, with "Elk Valley Springs" lettered on its front.

The uniformed guard looked up from his desk and sauntered out to meet me. "Hello, may I help you?"

"I'm here to see Blake Sagan."

His brows shot up briefly. "One moment, please." He returned to his post and, half a minute later, he spoke into the phone mouthpiece and chuckled.

"Mr. Sagan awaits," he called to me, apparently struggling to keep a straight face, and motioned me forward. "Enjoy your stay, Miss," he added with a wave, before he ducked back inside again.

Now the road curved upward in a graceful arc until it disappeared from sight between two hills. I drove over the top and caught my breath, then pulled off the road into a turnout to get a good look at the stunning panorama… and if I were honest, to compose myself.

View first.

I slid out of the seat and stumbled, legs half-numb from the drive, then took a deep breath and stretched my arms up over my head, my cramped muscles protesting at every movement.

Hawks played on the air currents high above Elk Valley as it spread out before me. Dark, pine-rimmed mountains encircling the tan, dry-grassed valley floor with occasional houses and small ranchettes around the perimeter. Other than the rustling in the dry scrub nearby, channeling images of rabbits and squirrels, the only other sound was the breeze whispering through the nearby pines. A taste of heaven for this country girl, especially after a month spent in the city.

Another big sigh.

What was I doing here, really?

My attention needed to be on my school, my career I'd pursued so diligently for all these years. Couldn't I wait?

Maybe he just wanted a friend…

Who are you kidding?

I screwed up my mouth and allowed myself a little grin.

No one.

With another deep inhalation, I climbed back into my car, no less resolved than I'd been upon my arrival at the gate.

A mile on, Prince stood in a field on my right, and I turned into the next driveway. Blake and the stallion stood silhouetted against a two-storied log cabin with dormer windows and a big, covered front porch. I shivered, shaken. Now was not the time to have my romantic dreams all come true at once. What the hell was I going to do with *this*?

I squelched the feelings and swallowed hard, then returned his wave, shifting my attention to the three dogs hurtling toward me from the front door of a barn on my right. Thankfully, they flowed around my old pickup as I continued up the drive, accompanied by Blake's futile shouts for them to leave off.

I parked in front of the house and schooled my face to neutral friendliness, but one glance in the rear-view mirror, showing Blake coming toward me, confirmed that yes, my cheeks were as red as they were hot.

Opening the door, I was attacked by three laughing dogs, with tongues lolling. I talked with them and tried to pet all three at once.

"Dogs, leave her alone!" Blake hustled up to save me.

"I was getting seriously concerned I might get licked to death," I told him as he gave me his hand and drew me from the cab of my truck into the middle of the melee.

"Welcome. So glad you could come." His smile went all the way to his eyes and there was little question he meant it with all his heart. "I'd like you to meet Jake LaRue Sagan, the boss."

I held a hand out to the gray-bearded Labrador and he planted a forefoot in it for a shake. The fat black dog beamed and shook for all he was worth, then came closer for a lick.

"And Kelpie Anne Sagan." Kelpie was, not surprisingly, a

red Kelpie. She wriggled around my legs and nearly knocked them out from under me. Solid, keen, and very friendly.

"And this little one is Sara Lee Sagan. She's the baby." The black and white cocker spaniel looked up at me with soft, sorrowful eyes and I stroked her head gently. Blake laughed. "She acts like a softie, but she sets these two back on their heels when her supper's threatened. She's just waitin' till your guard's down. She's a lot tougher than she looks."

"I'll be sure to watch her." I laughed, then glanced back down the drive to see Prince standing at attention. He called out to us in a loud, demanding, stallion-like voice.

"He wants you come down there, now, obviously, but you'll see him in a bit."

"Hello, Prince," I returned.

He shook his head, mane flying in all directions, and wandered away to pick at weeds in the dust of his pen.

"Can I get your bags? Then I'll show you upstairs."

"Yes, thank you." I smiled and handed him my overnight bag.

A gentleman. I could get used to this.

I told my insides to stop melting.

"Did you have a good drive up?" Blake led me toward the house.

"Beautiful," I sighed, gazing upward at the front of the cabin, with pretty calico curtains in the paned windows, "and you have a lovely home."

He winked at me. "Glad you like it. Took me years to build."

My jaw dropped. "You *built* it?" It was the biggest log cabin I'd ever seen, and the loveliest.

He nodded.

"Yourself?"

"Nope, Jake helped." He glanced at the grinning Labrador.

"Kelpie Anne tried, but she was just a pup—always in the way, and Sara Lee wasn't born yet."

I shook my head and gazed around as he led me into the house. The old-fashioned, floral pattern of the wallpaper complimented the mellowing pine of the trim and the rustic logs of the outer structural walls.

He was the perfect gentleman, but as he led the way upstairs, my heart was in my throat… I'd volunteered to come, but… like Ray said, I didn't know him from a bar of soap. Would he expect me to be staying in his room—his bed?

I swallowed hard and put my foot on the first step. I had a mouth, and I could say no, if I had to. Maybe this wasn't such a good idea, but now was a little late to be getting cold feet… wasn't it?

Stop being a fool and get on with it.

I took a deep breath as my fingertips slid smoothly along the hand-carved banister. I walked behind Blake, my heart squeezing tighter with every step upwards, then we were on a landing and he stood aside to let me precede him through a door into to a little room under the eaves. One look into the room and I let out the breath I'd been holding.

Its walls, with delicate cream flowers on a pale blue background, and the ruffled natural calico curtains framing the view of the mountains made me feel I'd just stepped into a fairy tale.

"It's beautiful," I breathed.

"Like it?" His smile stretched from ear to ear. "And out there," he pointed across the valley, "are trails around the whole valley."

My heart stopped for a moment. "Riding trails? Around the whole valley?" I flicked my gaze to his face and our eyes met.

He smiled and slowly nodded. "Ready to go for a ride?"

"We can go, now?" No five-year-old could have been more excited. I shook my head with a rueful smile at myself.

"Why do you think I invited you up here? You brought your riding gear, didn't you?"

My face flamed. He was being honorable and I'd just been thinking… no, better not to even think of that. I looked up and our eyes met. "Sure did. Breeches and boots okay?" I didn't think my grin could stretch any further. "You sure know how to make a girl happy."

"My specialty. Go change and I'll get drinks to take along."

I was ready in two minutes flat and met him outside in the brilliant mid-afternoon sunshine. As we turned the corner of the barn, a beautiful gray Arabian mare came into view.

"Her name is Miss Witeża, Tessa for short, Prince's wife. He adores her. They've had a few nice foals together, but they're still young yet."

"Are they here?"

"No, they've gone to good endurance homes."

Handing me a grooming kit and pointing out the mare's tack, he left me to make friends while I groomed and saddled her.

We mounted, and Blake pointed out the different trails around the valley while we rode down the drive and crossed the road circling the valley.

"It's too late for a long ride today, but I'll show you around what the brochures call *'the amenities Elk Valley Springs has to offer',*" he said, with a smarmy radio-announcer voice. "The fancy bits down here—the clubhouse, tennis courts, bar, gym —I don't use. I'm here for the dedicated horse trails and the fact I don't need to trailer to go for a good, long ride."

"If you're trying to convince me, you're wasting your breath. I saw all that when I topped the rise coming into the valley from the entrance gate. Oh, by the way, I was wondering something. The man at the entrance gate."

He grinned. "Yes? What about him? He's a friend of mine, of sorts…"

"Why the quirky smile on his face when he was speaking with you?"

"I told him quite some time ago that I was staying away from women. "

"So, why the grin?"

"You're a woman."

"And?"

He sighed and looked straight at me. "You're the first female younger than sixty-six who's arrived alone at that gate—looking for me—since I was married. A good six years ago."

My mouth opened, but nothing came out. I slapped it shut and bit my lips together. Not a playboy, then. That had to be good… I think.

But then, was I ready to try again?

BLAKE PULLED another piece of firewood from the basket beside the log wall and set it carefully on top of the already-stacked kindling in his wood stove.

Lena was a hoot. Not only that, she was a dream with the horses and dogs, and was simply… a pleasure to be around.

That doesn't mean I can trust her with my heart.

He lit the newspaper twists at the base of the stack, opened the flue and sat back.

That's probably never going to happen again.

Blake looked around and tugged the sheepskins off their stand and onto the floor in front of the fire, sat down on one, and leaned back against the sofa base.

Just what is my intent?

He wouldn't think of that for now. He planned every other part of his life to death. Maybe he could just let this one ride.

A board creaked on the stairway and Lena came into view, hair wet from her shower.

His intent got a little messed up, looking at her with her hair and her guard down. "Good shower?"

She smiled. "Good ride, good company, and a hot shower. What more could a girl want?"

"How about dinner before the fire?"

"Now you're talking." Her eyes lit up. "Can I help?"

"It's done. I hope you like steak and potatoes."

"Love them."

"Your steak?"

"Medium rare, please."

He grunted and headed to the kitchen. The barbecue out the back door was hot and ready to go. The steaks were ready in minutes and Blake returned with full plates to find her bent over, swinging her long hair before the fire to dry it. He gulped and nearly turned around. This "friendship" would get taxing if he had too many views like that. Clenching his jaw, he carried on and set their meals down on two trays.

"Already? You're quick."

"Quick, but not fast," Blake said, pleased she was now right side up with her bottom buried in the sheepskin.

Appetites piqued by their day in the sunshine, their meals disappeared in minutes, and Blake leaned back against the sofa again.

"So, what do you want to do tomorrow?" he asked.

"Whatever you need help with around here, and then maybe,"—she looked up at him with her big green eyes—"we could go for another ride."

"My kind of girl," he said, then clamped his jaw shut as his heart squeezed in his chest. He'd have to watch his mouth if he were—somehow—going to stay out of trouble.

But... why stay out of trouble?

Beside him, Lena lay back on the sheepskins, a sleepy smile on her face. So close. He could reach out and—

She leapt to her feet, terror in her eyes, then swallowed hard and looked at him.

He hadn't moved.

"Lena, what's the matter?"

She shook her head as the fear slowly melted from her visage and sat down again beside him, but a foot farther away. "It'll be okay," she murmured.

They were silent for long minutes, only the crackling of the fire and a dog snoring from its bed in the corner.

"Are you sure? Want to talk about it?"

She only shook her head in answer.

It clearly wasn't okay, but she wasn't talking about it tonight, that was for certain. "Where would you like to ride tomorrow?"

Her pale face was regaining some of its color and she made an attempt to smile as he told her of the trip around the rim to the south and west. He'd save the northern branch for her next visit.

It was special.

7

"And," I said to Raywyn as I sprayed the inside of the dog cage with disinfectant and climbed inside to wipe it down, which gave me time to think about how much I was going to tell her, "we spent the rest of the weekend sitting on Blake's front porch with the dogs, working with the horses, and riding."

"Riding?" The tone in Ray's voice was unmistakable, though it came from inside another kennel.

I shook my head, which of course, she couldn't see. "Riding *horses*, Ray. Get your mind out of the gutter. This guy isn't like all the college studs you keep telling me to avoid, my history notwithstanding. The man's a gentleman." I crawled out of the cage and reached for a stack of old newspapers.

"But what do you know about him?" She sat back on her heels, paper towels wadded up in one hand. "I mean, what do you really *know* about him? Is he some shyster on the make for a vet to support him? Criminal convictions? Is he an ax-murderer?"

I laughed outright and peeled off layers of newspaper to line the cage. "If you worried half as much about the men *you* find, I'd be happy. He's everything I've ever wanted: kind, loving, independent... I mean, you should see his eyes glow, and that smile... mmm."

"You're in trouble."

"He's gutsy, and he rides the stallion I adore." I hesitated, seeking just the right argument. "Okay, this should get you. Every animal I've ever seen him near adores him. His dogs have three names. Each."

Ray spun around, her eyes bugging. "Pardon?"

"You heard me." Smugly.

"Three?"

I told her. "And Jake LaRue Sagan helped him build his log cabin. They built it on their own."

Ray twisted her mouth and was silent.

"See? He's okay."

She drew in a big breath and let it out slowly. "That doesn't answer the question of his just looking for someone to support him. What does he do?"

"He's a short-haul pilot."

She blinked. "Really?"

I nodded and let a grin break through. Victory was sweet.

Ray must have been thinking hard. She was silent for long enough for me to clean, paper, and fleece three more cages while she finished one, and she was usually twice as fast as I was. "So, tell me about these horses," she said in quite a different voice.

I'm afraid I gushed, rather. "The horses are a hoot. Prince I've already told you about"—I smiled at her eye-rolling—"but he's so funny at home. When he's bored, he bites the near side of his feed bucket—one of those big, flat-bottomed rubber ones? Then he flips the thing over his head. He stands there, peering out from under it, his wild mane and forelock everywhere. When it finally falls off, he does it again and again until he finds something else to do."

"Those things weigh a ton," Ray said, with the first grin I'd seen on her face all morning.

"He's one strong boy. And the mare, Tessa, she's a Polish Arabian like Prince, but gray. Nearly as stocky as Prince, though. They're awesome horses. They both have Witez II for a grandsire, at least once."

"Isn't he that Polish Arabian stallion Patton's army rescued along with the Lippizaners during World War II?"

I nodded. "Disney made a movie about them. I loved it."

"Me too"—Ray raised a brow at me—"but you didn't ride horses all night, or maybe you di—"

"Ray," I cut in, "we very properly played Scrabble and chess in front of the firepl—"

"Excuse me, Ray," cut in Nancy, the receptionist. "We just had a cat come in. Can you please come check him out? Dr. Franco is on his way, but he'll be awhile."

"I'll be right there," Ray said. "We're done here, anyway. Let's go see this cat, but don't think"—she raised a suspicious brow at me and shook her head—"that you're getting off this lightly. I'm not done with you yet."

I laughed. "I hadn't imagined you were. Let's go see this cat."

OUR NEW PATIENT had to be one of the tallest cats I'd ever seen. Fred was a long, lean, and lanky gray two-year-old male. He looked far from all right, though, with the lower half of one hind leg from hock to toes lying flush with the examination table. His owners, a harried young couple with a herd of three under-fives, were in a panic.

"I've just lost my job." The young man flushed and swallowed hard. "And we have to move into an apartment… today."

They clearly loved the cat, and it was easy to see why. Despite the pain in his leg, he was still rubbing his head on the youngest child's grimy hand while another pulled lightly on his tail.

"I'm sure we can get him fixed up for you, but we'll have to wait for the vet. I'm only the vet student," I said, stroking the cat and surreptitiously picking up his paws one at a time. A gentle squeeze of the pads of his front feet showed his frayed claws—probably hit by car. "Is he an outside cat?" I asked, while I palpated the rest of his body with gentle touches of my fingers.

"Yes, we live—lived—a little way back from the road, but he's a bit of a wanderer," said the woman with a sad smile.

I'd seen it in textbooks, of course, the hock and metatarsals horizontal in the standing animal. Ruptured calcanean, or Achilles, tendon. The tendon had somehow been torn or else ripped off of the top of the calcaneus, analogous to our heel. It would require surgery, and not a minor one, at that. Fred seemed all right, otherwise. His color was fine and his heart and lungs sounded perfect.

"Problem is…"—the man went on, his knuckles white on the table—"or the problems are…. we can't keep him where we're going, and we've been trying to find him a new home… and… we don't have any money." He finished on a whisper and glanced at his children, his brow furrowed as he bit his lip.

I made comforting noises about the vet coming soon, but he stopped me.

"We have just enough to put him out of his pain."

I swallowed hard and clamped my jaw shut, trying not to let my feelings show. These people were barely hanging on, in more ways than one.

With only a surgery, this sweet and loving cat could live a long and happy life.

It's one of the hardest things about being a vet.

The choices are not always our own.

"I'm sorry," I said to Fred's owners, "but Dr. Franco won't be in for another hour. Do you have time to wait?"

The woman looked at her husband, then back at me. "We could run our errands and bring him back then, if it's all right with you."

"We'd be happy to keep him here for you, if you like," Raywyn said.

Her eyes lit up. "That would be very helpful," she murmured. "Thank you. We'll see you soon." She swallowed hard and kissed the cat on the head. "Come on, children, Fred's staying here but we'll return."

Fred's family came back half an hour after the vet arrived and waited for the doctor in the reception area. By then, Dr. Franco, or James, as I'd known him since I was a child, had caught up with the already-accumulated backlog of patients. I cornered him before he went out to see Fred's owners.

"You can't save everything, Lena." The vet closed his eyes, then opened them and looked hard at me. "And this is no exception."

"But look at him. He's a fantastic cat.... loving, kind, and so *young*."

"They want him euthanized."

"They don't want him euthanized, but they don't have the money to have the surgery... and they can't keep him."

He glanced up from the gray beast rubbing his head on his hand to see the hopeful look on Ray's face and then his eyes narrowed at me. "What have you two been cooking up?"

"Well..." I couldn't help wincing. "We—"

"Don't get *me* into trouble, Lena. It was *you* who cooked up this hare-brained scheme," Ray cut in.

"*I* thought," I corrected, "maybe if I did the surgery and paid for the materials and drugs, I could find him a home... that is, if the owners agree."

He rubbed his hands over his eyes, silent for a moment.

"It'd be... in the interest of my training." I said, in a rush. Not the truth, but if the shoe fits...

He took a deep breath and let it out slowly, then raised a brow at me. "You're determined to save him, aren't you?"

"He's such a lovely cat. You should have seen him with his children. This cat deserves to live."

James considered for a minute, then shook his head with a rueful smile. "Okay, if they agree to sign him over and you can find him a home this week, we can do this. And," grudgingly, "you won't be paying me anything. You're more than earning your keep."

I hugged him and raced from the room.

"The doctor will see you now," I said to the family, somehow stifling the whoop that begged to be let out. They filed silently into the room and flocked around the gray ball of fluff Ray held on the table.

When Dr. Franco explained the offer, both adults burst into tears and agreed with everything. They signed on the dotted line with watery smiles and I was now the proud owner of a very large, loving, cat. Now I just needed to do a good job of the surgery... and find him a home.

The cat's previous family left, planning to return to visit him after his surgery. They were sad to be losing him, but happy he could have the life they could no longer offer.

My heart swelled that we could give them and the gray cat some happiness, but my happiness was shadowed by thoughts of all the other animals in similar situations... who didn't get this option.

As it turned out, we had time to do the surgery the same afternoon Fred was left with us.

My heart squeezed tight in my chest at the thought of performing this surgery on my own as I pored over the surgery textbooks on the practice library's shelves. I made notes and drew diagrams of different options, depending upon what we found on X-rays and further examination, to lash the tendon back in place. I finished with a surgical plan for James' approval.

"What's your first step?" the vet said and took a bite of his ham and Swiss on rye.

"Radiograph the leg."

"Looking for…?" he said after he'd finished chewing.

"Determine whether it's a simple gastrocnemius tendon rupture or an avulsion fracture of the end of the tuber calcanei." I popped the last bite of donut, not an ideal lunch, into my mouth and awaited his next question. Despite being quizzed, lunchtime discussions were less stressful than vet school pre-surgery rounds.

"Good. And if it's a tendon rupture or an avulsion fracture?"

"Surgery as soon as possible, before the tendon has a chance to shorten. If it's a tendon tear alone, suture with polypropylene in a Bunnell pattern."

"How likely is a pure tendon rupture in the absence of a wound?"

"Unlikely. It's probably a chip or avulsion fracture, though I suspect he's been hit by a car, so it could be anything. With his youth and large size, I'd be looking for an epiphyseal avulsion—separation at the growth plate. I'd repair that with 4-0 stainless steel in a Bunnell pattern again, and… let's hope it's just a chip fracture and not the epiphysis, then we can just fix the tendon to the remainder of the calcaneus, and pins and tension band wire won't be needed, as they would if the growth plate has been pulled off."

"Very nice. Good plan. We'll make a small animal vet out of you yet," he said, and stood up from the lunchroom table. "Let's take those films."

While I slid the cassette beneath the lounging cat, my mind was ticking over. I could keep Fred, but what to do with him until I returned home?

Cats can be tricky to X-ray, but not Fred.

"Here?" he seemed to say, when I positioned him. He must've meant, "I like the feel of that sandbag on top of one leg and under the other," by the purrs vibrating through the table.

"What a cat," I said, to James. "You can leave, I've got this. He's not going anywhere." As soon as he cleared the room, I started up the rotor and clicked the button.

"All clear," I called, and he returned.

"You're right, that cat's really somethin'. Let's just start with that one before we try for an AP."

I smiled smugly and took the cassette and label into the developing room, locked the door, reached for the developing frame by rote and set it down before me. I checked for light leaks around the door while my eyes adjusted to the red light in the room's dark interior, then snapped open the cassette. Carefully removing the film, I clicked it in the labeler and scrabbled for the almost-invisible steel frame. After manhandling the film into the frame, I dropped it into the first tank and gave it a swirl, then refilled the cassette with a fresh film.

"I can take over here," Ray called through the door.

"Ok, let me get the lids on and it's all yours."

"Thanks, Ray," I said a few moments later as I exited, blinking in the brightness. "It's just gone into the developer and the timer's set.

"I'll be out to do Fred's anesthesia in a few minutes," she said with a smile, and sent me on my way.

Ray had already set up for his surgery, bless her soul. The unopened sterile pack, scrub kit, drapes, gowns, and gloves lay neatly on the trolley in the scrub room adjacent to the surgical suite.

I'm glad the surgery was today, so I didn't have too much time to think about the effect this surgery could have on Fred's life.

The x-ray was perfect. Even better, it showed no displaced piece of bone, indicating it was just a rupture of the tendon itself.

With James, silent on the opposite side of the surgical field, acting as my vet technician, the procedure went like clockwork. The polypropylene behaved and knotted only when I wanted it to, and the injury must've happened just before they brought him in, because I was able to draw the long fragment of the gastroc tendon down and reattach it to its partner with a minimum of fuss.

Before Fred woke up, we placed a splint on the leg to keep him from tearing our work apart before it healed. It would take some time—tendon healing is slow.

"Now you just need to find him a home," James said, later that afternoon.

"I'm working on it," I said. "And James, thanks for giving him, and me, a chance."

"I'm not as crusty as I want people to think," he said and ruffled my hair as he left for the day.

Ray saw the exchange and watched the vet walk out the front door. "He could be up for harassment with that."

"It's okay. I've known him and whole family since I was little. They lived next door while he was an undergraduate student at Stanford."

"Really? I didn't know that."

"Yep. I tagged along with him on our 'fix the neighborhood animals' rounds when I couldn't have been more than seven or eight. When he moved on to veterinary school, I took over his rounds."

"You've wanted to do this for a long time," Ray shook her head.

I nodded and raised my brows at her. "Well, what's left to do? I've cleaned all the instruments and have a hankering to clean some kennels and go home."

"You're on. Besides, I have more questions for you."

I smiled. "Hey, you know, small animal medicine isn't so bad. I could get to like it."

"Doing surgery usually turns people around. Either you love it or you hate it. You did a great job today."

"It helped that I don't seem to be allergic to Fred."

Ray laughed.

"And your anesthesia, as always, was perfect. I hope someday I'll find a vet tech as good as you." Ray really was good at what she did and I appreciated her no end.

"So, when are you"—Ray handed me a bucket of cleaning materials and turned toward the kennels—"going to hear from him again?"

"Probably… on Friday night."

"He's calling you then?"

"Ah… no. I'm going back."

8

"Back." Ray turned away from the row of cages in the kennel to face me, hand on hip. "You're going back there already?"

I looked at her sideways. "Something wrong with that?"

"You just met the guy. He's going to think you're too eager and drop you."

"I *am* eager"—I twisted my lips for a moment—"but trying not to look like it."

"And going up to his place again isn't eager?"

"Look, Ray, I love that he lives in a beautiful place, that he has a career that lets him train and compete his horses, that he's excited about my becoming a vet, and most of all, that he's a genuinely nice guy who had me in his home for the entire weekend—and didn't try to jump my bones. If that's not a match made in heaven, I don't know what is."

"I just"—Ray scrubbed her fingers through her hair—"don't want to see you get hurt."

"Tell me about it. I don't either." I gave her a sheepish grin. "Thanks for giving a damn."

She shook her head, then turned toward the first cage, armed with her spray bottle of disinfectant.

"Anyway, I have to go see my mom," I said.

"But she lives up north, doesn't she?"

"Not anymore. She's halfway between here and Blake's, in a roundabout fashion. I miss her—I haven't seen her since Christmas. It'll be nice to see her."

Nice, as long as she doesn't hear about Blake.

"I'm not sure how that guy managed to get her in here," I said, absently stroking the Irish Setter's long, soft ears as James and I sat by the red dog's cage late on Wednesday night. "He carried her five blocks after he saw that car hit her."

I'd come downstairs to help James when the emergency call came in and had met the man at the front door.

"He'd had a few too many," James said, with a smile.

"He was potted, all right," I said.

The vet smiled. "And she isn't even his dog." He adjusted the drip and lifted the bitch's lip to check her color again, then looked at me. "It's a bit like old times," he said.

"From the emergency clinic?"

He nodded, with a smile.

"Good thing you and your wife talked me back into aiming for vet school after my ridiculous high school counselor told me it was 'hard to get into vet school and maybe I should think of something else'." I finished on a growl.

"Idiot. She should've known better. You had the highest GPA in your high school, played in band, did cheerleading and pom pom, rode that big chestnut horse of yours, worked part time, and graduated a full year early."

"I'm going back to visit her someday. I promise you, she won't do *that* again."

He laughed. "And when you first found us down here, you were studying English, history and Spanish at the UC."

"Complete with a humanities student's fear of science, by then."

"But you took that job in my emergency clinic and studied hard, and now you're in vet school." He smiled at me. "But I was thinking about the bar next door to the emergency clinic."

I snorted. "The customers always peered in the front windows when the bar closed at two. I'd be alone there, scrubbing floors," I said, with a shudder. "I'd always leave the back rooms for their closing time, so I could hide. And then the phone would start to ring. All emergencies, whatever the problem."

"Drunk callers." He shook his head with a rueful grin.

"Good thing they didn't tend to show up," I said, with a smile. "You'd never have gotten *any* sleep." I returned my attention to the setter's silky coat. "Thanks for taking her in. You probably won't get paid for this one, you know."

"Has that stopped me before?"

"Nope," I smiled, "it sure hasn't. And you've been a good role model. Thanks, James."

SARAH, the part-time receptionist, put her head around the door into the treatment room early the next morning. "Lena, has Dr. Franco arrived yet?"

"No, sorry, he hasn't." I gave the countertop a final swipe with the cloth. "Is there an emergency?"

"Well, sort of," she said, and bit her lip. "Shall I show them into the exam room?"

"Yes, thanks. I'll come take a look."

A few minutes later I stopped just outside the exam room and froze. Whatever it was, it was quite possibly demonic. I waved Ray over to listen.

"Do you want to go in there or shall I?" I whispered.

"It might take two of us." Ray glared at the door. "Dr. Franco keeps promising to put a peephole into this door." She took a deep breath and opened it just a crack, then held it open for me. The beast must be securely contained.

I peered into the room. A plastic cat cage sat on the floor beside the feet of a tousled young man. I use the term "sat" loosely. Very loosely.

The container was doing anything but sitting. It bumped from side to side. It even bounced a little. From the howls and yowls, I assumed it was a cat. Frankly, I wasn't game to duck down and have a good look until I needed to.

With an apologetic look upon his face, the young man stood and offered a scratched and bleeding hand for me to shake. "Thomas. Thank you, Doctor, for seeing me so quickly. I hit it"—he nodded at the dancing cat carrier—"with my car." He shrugged. "I couldn't leave it there by the side of the road."

A heinous combination of a growl and a hiss came from the box. Something I'd expect from a rather pissed-off tiger.

"Can you please put the cage onto the examination table?" I said, then flinched as a ginger claw shot out and sank into the hand he was using to steady the carrier while he lifted it with the other.

With amazing presence of mind, Thomas somehow got the cat's nails out of his hand without shrieking or dropping the plastic handle and set the semi-contained beast on the table. He did leap away, however, when the cat's paw hooked the wire front door and yanked several times, threatening to tear it from its mounting and decapitate everyone in the room.

An eerie howl filled the room as we all took a step back from the hidden monster.

"Thank you for bringing him in." Ray ducked down to peek into the cat box but didn't get too close. "Or her, as the case may be. Is this your cat?"

"No," he said. "I've never seen it before. It's got to be the biggest cat I've ever seen. Do you think it's a Maine Coon? I've always wanted one."

"Hard to say," Ray raised a brow and shook her head at me behind the excited young man's back.

"The receptionist had me fill out my details," he said helpfully, and straightened up. "She left it on the countertop over there." He pointed.

"So she did, thanks." I took it up and glanced at the neat lettering. "*Stray HBC*".

"When was he hit by the car?" I asked.

He glanced at his watch, which was smeared liberally with blood. "Half an hour ago."

"How did you get him into the cage? He doesn't seem very happy in there." Ray commented, keeping her distance while trying to see the animal in the dark interior.

"He was pretty out of it. I carried him home. He just woke up on the way here. He's been yowling ever since. Do you think he'll be all right?"

"I'm just the student," I said, thanking my lucky stars. "We'll have to wait until the vet gets here to do a full exam. Thanks so much for bringing him in."

"Of course. Couldn't do anything else, right?" He gave me an anxious glance.

"We have your information, so you don't have to wait."

"I'm headed for work, but I can come get him on the way home. Just before five?"

"Does he have a collar on or anything? Anything to

identify him?" Ray said, her eyebrows nearly touching her hairline.

He shook his head. "No, sorry."

"It's okay. SPCA will come pick him up, so you needn't worry about him anymore. It was really nice of you to bring him in."

He gave me a horrified look. "I hit him, I'll take full responsibility. And I'll come get him tonight. He might belong to one of my neighbors."

I shot him a sideways glance, which he thankfully missed.

He wanted to take that *home?*

Ten minutes later, Thomas stepped out the front door, his wounds cleansed, disinfected, and bandaged in the back room to the accompaniment of Ray's admonitions about tetanus vaccination and cat scratch fever. "Look at it this way," she said, "maybe the cat just hates the carrier. I'm sure he'll be fine once he gets out."

"Out?" I stared at her blankly. The only "out" I could see for that cat was general anesthesia. This was one of those days I was glad to be the student, and not the vet.

It was an eventful morning, and I counted myself truly blessed to see just what a true master of a vet and a gem of a vet tech could do together to get that—wild—cat out of the cage and into an anesthetic induction chamber to repair the lacerations on two of its legs.

"I'm only thankful for absorbable sutures and that we don't have to do bandage changes," I said with a shudder. "Do you think he's truly wild?"

Ray nodded. "No doubt about it. I'm not sure what Thomas is going to do with him."

Just before five, the sleeping cat lay oblivious in the cat carrier as Thomas carried him out of the clinic.

"Thank you so much," he turned in the doorway to beam at us. "I was so upset when I thought I'd killed him."

"Are you sure you don't want SPCA to come pick him up? We think he's truly wild," Ray said.

"No, we'll be fine," he said, smiling. "I think I'll call him George."

I winced. "Please take care. I'd hate to see you even more scratched up."

"I think we'll be fine," he said, and he walked out the door.

We both waved at his back as he disappeared around the corner.

I looked at Ray, who was still waving. "Promise me," I said to her, "if we read of his death by cat scratch fever at the hands of a cross between a rabid Honey Badger and a cat, you'll go with me to the funeral."

She took my hands in hers and nodded solemnly. "But we won't be searching the papers too hard," she said and shuddered.

On Friday evening when I drove up in front of the log cabin, Blake looked as happy to see me as the dogs were... and that was saying a lot. He took my hand to help me out of the pickup as if I were a princess.

I could really get used to this.

"Hard week?" He leaned toward me, then swallowed hard and straightened up.

I pretended not to notice.

Blake reached for my bag and led me toward the house.

"Busy, but good." I hesitated for a moment, then asked the all-important question. "Blake, do you like... cats?"

"Yeah, why?"

While we headed up the stairs, I told him Fred's story.

"Can't wait to see him. He sounds like one cool cat. 'Fred'.

Even his name sounds like he's a character." Blake grinned as he set my suitcase on the bed in my little room under the eaves.

"He's been keeping us entertained in the treatment room when we let him out for some exercise. Talks up a blue streak."

"If you love him that much already, he's welcome to live here, no problem." Blake's eyes were warm on my face.

"So, that's me unpacked." I glanced out the window at the sun-kissed valley. "What's next? Ride? Feed?"

"It's a little late to ride and the feeding's all done, but nachos went into the oven when the dogs went nuts at your arrival. We just have time to go say goodnight to the horses before the cheese melts."

The dogs started barking again outside and I looked out the window to see a pickup with a vet pack on the back revving its way up the drive. "It's a vet."

"It's Doc Latimer." Blake took the stairs two at a time, with a glance out the stairwell window. "Jake might lick him to death. Best we go save him."

"Where's his practice?" Lena asked.

"It's down in Inyokern. I talked with him the other day and he said he'd come by if he was up here."

Blake dragged the dogs off of his legs. For a vet, dogs sure loved him.

"Good to meet you, Lena, call me Seth."

"Okay, Seth."

"I hear you've only got two years left at school." Seth smiled.

Lena nodded. "Seems like forever, but I'm sure it'll feel like the blink of an eye when I don't have anyone to hold my hand anymore when I'm out in practice."

"You got that right"—he laughed—"but hopefully you'll get a good boss to guide you along."

"I'm aiming for that, sir."

"So, Seth"—Blake looked at him sideways—"you wouldn't still be looking for a vet up this way, would you?"

"I just might be." Seth smiled at Lena. "Especially since I hear there's an up and coming equine track student who's been hanging around the valley."

Lena shot a look at Blake. Surprised, yes, but was she pleased or annoyed? She turned back to Seth, her back a little stiffer than usual.

Hard to tell.

Blake hoped she was happy about it, because right or wrong, and most likely too soon, he was already getting used to the idea of Lena in his life.

Seth must've noticed, because he changed the subject, asking if certain of the vet school instructors were still there. "Seriously? Old Lucas is still in charge of the barns? He was there when I was a student!"

"He's still my favorite out there. That man's full of knowledge." Lena was smiling again, and Blake breathed a sigh of relief.

"Seth, will you stay for some nachos?" he asked. "Speaking of which—" he dashed back into the house and rescued the only slightly over-browned platter.

"Sorry, Blake," Seth said when Blake returned. "But I've got to get a move on. We have company for dinner tonight, but another time soon? Lena, I look forward to seeing you again. Come on by for dinner when you're down our way."

"I know that one"—Blake laughed—"but you're never there. We'll take our chances of seeing you up here."

"Smart man," Seth said, and tipped his hat at Lena. "Ma'am."

The dogs trailed him to the truck and gazed at him

mournfully as he closed the door and waved, then headed down the drive.

The nachos were good, and the dogs soon forgot their favorite vet was gone, wriggling and grinning ingratiatingly beneath their feet at the big picnic table on the deck.

I AWOKE to the sun through the windowpanes etching a lattice pattern over the profusion of tiny white flowers on the wall and stretched. Even this single bed was heavenly after sleeping on a sofa bed for a month in Ray's apartment over the clinic.

Blake's voice came from outside and I peeked over the window sill. The dogs ran from the far side of the field toward him, where he was grooming the mare. Was it still ogling when you gazed upon a man in a skin-tight tank top out the window of his own house? My face warmed at the thought.

I dressed and looked out the window again.

Blake turned and looked up toward my window. He must've seen me then, and he waved.

I opened the casement and leaned out, hoping the cool air would do its job on my face. "Good morning! I'll be right down."

"No rush," he called and resumed his efforts to make Tessa's coat look something closer to its normal gray, and not dust-brown.

"What are you up to in here?" Blake said, when he found me in the kitchen a short time later.

"I brought breakfast, seeing as you've been spoiling me so much."

"What is it?" he said, peeking over my shoulder as I broke eggs into a bowl.

"Cottage cheese pancakes. Nearly 100% protein." Cottage cheese and a handful of flour followed, plus a pinch of salt, then I whizzed them with my stick blender. "Bacon's nearly done out on the barbecue, and I'm ready to do the pancakes on the griddle."

"Home-cooked breakfast"—he beamed—"and the eggs are already in it."

Blake loved them, especially when I brought out the applesauce.

"I could get used to this," he said, leaning back and taking a deep breath. "There's no room for more, and those were great, thanks. Are you ready to ride?"

"As ever." I hopped up.

"How about you get your gears on? I'll throw these in the dishwasher and pack us a snack," Blake threw over his shoulder as he and our plates disappeared toward the kitchen.

Blake's humming wafted up the stairs as he tinkered in the kitchen while I dropped my shorts and tugged on breeches and boots, then raced down the steps two at a time until I came up short before an older woman standing at the foot of the stairs.

"Oh, hello," I said, shrinking a bit at the disapproving look she aimed at my form-fitting breeches.

She pursed her lips and glanced up at my face but didn't say a word.

9

The humming from the kitchen ceased and Blake stuck his head around the corner. "Oh, I see you've met Myrtle." He looked sideways at the woman. "Myrtle," he said, "this is Lena. She's here for the weekend."

"Oh," she said, and the corners of her lips turned up in a caricature of a smile in my direction. "Hello," she said to me, then turned back to Blake with a beatific smile. "I was just about to put your dinner on."

Blake blinked. "As I said yesterday, that won't be necessary, thanks. Lena and I will be out for dinner."

Now it was Myrtle's and my turn to blink. Blake hadn't said anything to me about wining and dining. I'd have so set some boundaries.

Like you're setting boundaries now? Spending another weekend with a man you don't even know… and you're worried about a dinner date and a two-legged watchdog?

"You ready?" Blake glanced at me and hefted a set of full

saddlebags over his shoulder. He held the door open, said goodbye to Myrtle, and ushered me out and down the driveway toward the barn.

I held my silence, wondering just who Myrtle was.

I didn't have long to wait.

"Oh, and about Myrtle, don't worry about her. She's just a boarder, but she takes good care of the animals when I'm away."

"She lives with you all the time?" I didn't think I acted surprised, but must have, because he laughed.

"Yes. She was away visiting her daughter last weekend, so you didn't meet her before. Myrtle thinks she needs to guard me against all comers, but she's all right. And the dogs love her."

"A lot to be said for that." With a lighter heart, I beamed in his direction. Spending time with this pleasure of a man and horses *too*...

"Trees or wide-open spaces?" he asked, pointing one way and then the other. "Your choice."

"Trees, most definitely."

"Your wish is my command, milady." He grinned and turned Prince toward a thick belt of pines running along the base of the steep mountains rising from the valley floor. "This trail circles the whole valley and meets up with the trail we took last weekend."

I stared around the perimeter. "That's got to be fifty or sixty miles!"

"Sure is, fifty miles of dedicated horse trails. That's why we can hold our fifty-miler here."

"Here? An endurance ride?"

"Yep, later in the year, or rather, early next."

"What a place to live," I breathed. What I wouldn't give to live in a place with this sort of riding... it'd been my dream forever.

Blake glanced at my face and nodded, as his smile grew. "Yep, it's always been my dream, too," he said, as if reading my mind. "That's why I bought land here."

I shook my head, gazing around.

Heaven to a horsey-girl.

"So, I get to ride and train these horses three days a week." He gazed off into the distance. "Life doesn't get much better."

"I'd say it wouldn't," I said with feeling, then glanced his way. "Three days a week? How do you manage that?"

He gave me a cheeky grin. "I was fed up with trying to get two horses fit to race on two days a week. It was okay before, when I was marrie—" Blake stopped like he'd been shot, his visage masked for a moment. "Doing it on my own was too hard," he resumed smoothly. It took all the pleasure out of it. What's life for, if you spend your whole life working and don't take any time to enjoy it?"

"I understand," I murmured, though at my current position in life, I lived with constant work—every day.

"So, I told my boss I was going to quit, retire early."

"Just like that?" I stared at him, a sinking feeling in my chest. Security issues panicked me.

"Just like that."

"And… what did you do?

"I guess when you've been flying for a company for as long as I have, they get used to having you around. He wanted me to stay and asked what I wanted. I told him I wanted a four-day work week and no overnight trips away."

"And they bought it." It was a statement, rather than a question.

"Sure did. And they gave me a raise." He quirked his mustache.

"Well done," I said, with a chuckle, as I guided the mare between some rocks. I needn't have bothered, she knew this trail better than I ever would. I stroked her shiny neck. "Tessa's lovely. Never puts a foot wrong, does she?"

Blake shook his head. "Nope. She's amazing, and you ride her well. She's happy with you up there."

My heart glowed. There was no finer praise from a horseman of Blake's caliber. Riding partner he may be, but something inside me was liking the sound of Blake… probably too much.

We'd been riding for a few hours, alternating walking and trotting through treed gullies and open hillsides of low brush and rock, keeping an eye out for rattlesnakes, when Blake indicated a rise up ahead.

"Just up there," he said.

"What is it?"

"My picnic ground," he said, his eyes shining. "Nobody's usually up here, so we should have the place to ourselves."

Sounded fine to me. We walked the last mile and by the time we got to the spot, marked by a tinkling stream running delicately past it, the horses were completely cool and dry. A thick cushion of pine needles dampened the sound of the horses' hooves as we rode off the trail and stopped beneath the overhanging branches.

After we dismounted and unsaddled, Blake pulled out halters, leads, and a picket line, which I helped him fix between two trees.

"If you want to water them, I'll get our meal out."

"Sounds fine," I said and took Prince's lead from him, pleased the mare wasn't on heat and once again grateful Prince was such a well-behaved stallion. The sharp, astringent scent of pine needles crunching underfoot filled my nostrils as I led the horses to drink, then tied them both to the picket line.

Turning away from the horses, I filled my lungs and finally looked down the hill at the view. It took my breath away. Our other rides had mostly been down on the flats or in the lower slopes of the hills encircling the valley. We'd climbed so gradually I'd barely noticed the change in elevation, but now I saw how high we'd come. Elk Valley spread out before us. It was similar to the panorama I'd seen from near the entrance gates, but from this height, everything was spread out and so much clearer. The ring road, flanked by occasional houses with their own barns and corrals, surrounded a central cluster of buildings and several arenas. Higher up, stands of pines topped the high ridges surrounding the valley, continuous with the one in which I now stood. One last look and I turned back to where Blake had already set out his "snack".

"When you said"—I sank down onto the forest cushion beside him on an actual *tablecloth*, wincing as my abused muscles contacted the ground—"you were bringing a snack, I thought cheese and crackers and a beer, or something…"

He grinned with triumph across the tablecloth. Blake knew how to make friends. Out of the saddlebags had come a sumptuous meal. Succulent chicken, ham, cheeses, sourdough French bread, and wonder of wonders, a *salad*.

"How"—I shook my head, staring at the veritable feast—"did you manage to get all of this here in one piece, much less a salad?" The crispy greens and tomatoes were in perfect condition. "I couldn't manage that in my kitchen, and this has travelled for two hours on a trotting horse."

He laughed. "Magic, I guess. I've been packing a long time. It grows on you."

By the time our hunger was sated, I was starting to stiffen up. I'd barely ridden, even on my own horse, in six months and while it didn't affect my riding ability, my muscles weren't used to it. Tomorrow would be hellish, and I wouldn't let myself even consider how I'd feel the following day. The horses, however, were fine. Used to this life, they'd nibbled what wisps of grass they could reach, then dozed, one hind leg cocked, tails lazily swishing at the ever-present flies, while Blake pointed out more trails and landmarks.

The ride, the sun, the horses... and the man. Kind, generous, keen to share his time and place with me, and handsome—summed up, it was deadly... and downright sexy. Along with the good Danish Blue and Swiss on delicate, fragile (how *did* he do it?) crackers, the combination was a heady mix and I feared if I looked into his eyes, he'd see how affected I was. And that was far, far away from even resembling a good idea. I had goals... and dreams... but the hard edges around these seemed to be softening.

I lay back and covered my eyes with one arm, hiding. A few minutes later, I sighed and sat up. "I can't imagine a more perfect place to live with your horses. Nice and quiet. Just the way I like it."

"Yeah, well, it's quiet," he said. "I hadn't meant to live all al—" he broke off, his jaw set.

I turned away to give him some space in the pregnant silence.

"Dessert," he announced with a quick sigh and the flash of a grin I was coming to love.

"Thanks for inviting me," I said, then blinked as he spooned whipped cream onto one side of a bowl packed full of dark chocolate-dipped strawberries. I stared, open-mouthed, at the extravagance, then frowned at him. "This was not an impromptu lunch you whipped up this morning."

"Ya think?" He handed me the bowl, one eyebrow raised.

"I *know*. This was premeditated." I accepted the bowl with a smile. The man might have ulterior motives, but I couldn't blame him. My resolves were slipping further and further by the wayside.

"I aim to please, ma'am." He smiled off into the distance for a moment, then turned back to me. "I *do* plan—I can't help myself. Remember, I'm a pilot. But... this is just what I'd do for a friend."

I doubted the latter, but who was I to look a gift horse in the mouth when he was such a stunning specimen? I tried to tell myself I was just thinking of Prince, but even I wasn't fooled.

I handed the bowl back. Even before our fingers touched, the surge of something—electricity? —between us made me shiver. "Static," I said, shakily.

"Mmm..." he said, with a glance at me as he took a strawberry from the bowl. He hesitated, his hand straying toward me, as if he'd offer me a bite, then with a little shake of his head, lowered his arm and took a bite of it himself, his attention locked on the gilded fruit.

I swallowed hard. I'm afraid I'd have accepted the proffered bite from his fingers, if he'd continued. I was starting to think those resolutions of mine might be silly, after all.

"They're filled," Blake said, just as the sweet almond scent hit me.

My teeth sank into the crimson flesh and chocolate melded with amaretto to send my already-heightened senses skyrocketing. Damn good thing he hadn't offered me a bite of his strawberry; I'd probably be in his lap by now.

Get your mind out of the gutter, girl!

I straightened my spine. "How'd you get the chocolate to stick?" was the first thing that fell out of my mouth. It stopped us both, anyway.

He chuckled. His voice rumbled deeper than I'd ever heard it, or was I just on another planet?

"Dip them first, then inject them with amaretto after the chocolate has set."

My mouth formed a silent "O" as I nodded, and Blake gazed across at me.

"Of course. The amaretto would leak out all of the little

pinholes in the berry's surface. I haven't tried making them," I rambled at random, "but my sister complained she couldn't get the chocolate to stick. I'll definitely make them now." I fumbled for something witty to say—and failed, then tried to think about something... something safe... *anything* other than the thought of Blake's strong fingers molded around a big, luscious strawberry, feeding the chocolatey goodness to me, then tracing a line down my throat—

Stop it!

There were far too many deep sighs coming from my direction. It was high time for desperate measures. If my brain wouldn't work, maybe my body would. I jumped to my feet. "So, the trail, it goes right the way around?" I said, my voice too deep for the question.

Blake smiled up at me lazily from his horizontal position, lying back with his folded arms for a pillow. A fleeting glance at his jeans told me he wasn't as unaffected as he seemed. I shook my head and shut my eyes for a moment. He just controlled himself better than I did.

A thought finally flashed through my brain. "Did you do all this?" I pointed at the closed, empty containers, "or Myrtle?"

He sent me a smug grin. "It was all me. Myrtle'd like to mother me, or worse, get me to think she's thirty years younger and marry me, but it just ain't gonna happen. She likes to throw her weight around when there are other women around. I don't think she wants her place here threatened, but as I said"—he twisted his lips—"I can't do this alone with the horses and the dogs." He filled his lungs and breathed out slowly. "So it works, for now."

I smiled down at him. "I'm glad you're making it work."

"Me too." He heaved a great sigh. "Things are about to get even busier with the ride we're running in January."

"Oh yeah." I blinked. "In the winter?"

Blake gave a short laugh. "Remember? We're in the high desert." He scraped free a little of the gritty soil from beneath the pine needles and let it run through his fingers. "It doesn't rain much, so conditions up here are perfect for a post-Christmas ride." He turned those gorgeous baby blues straight into mine. "You should come down."

I think I sputtered something about clinic rotations or some such nonsense and he cocked a brow at me.

"Just after Christmas? Cripes, girl, they need to let you have *some* time off."

"Oh, they do… it's just…" I floundered, but I finally couldn't help letting a smile break through. I took a deep breath. "Frankly, I probably won't have the money. I barely make enough to feed my horse, the cat, and me."

He looked at me sideways. "You forget. I'm a pilot, and we fly into Sacramento."

My face heated. This man didn't just think of getting his rocks off for today. January was half a *year* away. I gulped and sat down beside him again. The thought was terrifying, but somehow, despite the barriers I'd so carefully built, it was also comforting. "I'd like that," I said, with caution. "Let's see how we go."

"Another strawberry?" His voice was slow, deep, and syrupy, like the chocolate he'd nearly tried to feed me before.

Something tightened down deep inside me at his words and I looked up to see him holding the largest, most beautiful berry in his fingers. Its surface glistening with droplets of liqueur and capped with brown gold, he held it up this time toward my lips, and in his intent gaze lingered an expectancy.

10

I swallowed hard as Blake moved the gilded strawberry toward my lips. I froze, then slowly opened my mouth to accept the fruit and bit down. The juicy, aromatic goodness melted into my mouth, and we both laughed as the amaretto dribbled down my chin. As one, we reached to catch the drips before they hit my shirt, our fingers colliding in a tangle.

With a sharp inhalation, Blake sat back and handed me the rest of the berry, his face as flushed as mine no doubt was.

I took a shaky breath, along with the stem of the strawberry, and focused my attention on it.

Neither of us was unaffected. That was patently obvious now.

But where to go or not to go?

That was the question.

Somehow, we fumbled our way through packing up our lunch and mounting up again.

Once we were safely on the trail, I dared to look at Blake. Our eyes met, then slid away again. Best take the bull by the horns here.

"That was a wonderful lunch, thank you, and especially—" my gaze lifted to his face, "—dessert."

The tight lines around his mouth melted a little and he smiled. "Liked that, did you?" His Adam's apple bobbed a few times, then he reached forward to stroke the stallion's neck.

He did that a lot, the stroking.

I think I might be starting to get a little jealous.

I snorted and attempted to change the circular track beginning to wear its way around my brain. "So, how long will the ride be, the January one?"

The tension in his hands upon the reins, the only place I dared to look, softened, and a look of excitement replaced doubt. "It's a fifty-miler. We're not having a twenty-five, don't want to mess with people who don't bother to train for it, then use up all our resources because their horse crashes. We're light on vets around here and we need them to take care of all the horses, not just the unfit, crashing ones. It's only fair."

"Good thinking. It'd sure be nice to come down."

"Keep it in mind. I can get you a cheap flight. They might let you fly jump-seat, if I ask the right person."

I grinned. This could be a fun friendship.

Friendship, ha. We'll see how long it stays at that.

I shook my head to clear it.

"You know"—he flicked me a glance—"we *are* short on good horse vets in this valley."

"Don't tempt me. My uncle's already put in his dibs. He wants my help on his stud farm and he's dangling carrots, like an on-site clinic."

Blake's brows shot up. "Generous offer."

Tessa stopped short, her body rigid. I swung around to face forward... toward the yawning gap in the trail not two yards ahead of her planted forefeet.

"Good girl, Tess," I murmured, and slowly backed the mare, afraid our movements might let even more of the trail slip away, taking us with it.

I stared across the gap of nearly six yards-worth of trail. A massive pile of dirt and rubble—the remains of the trail—rested in the valley far below.

"What is it?" Blake barked from his position behind us.

"There's a landslide up here. Looks like a new one," I threw over my shoulder, my voice and the rest of me shaking, and kept backing the mare until I was level with Prince.

I slid to the ground and into Blake's arms. "That was close," I mumbled into his shirt front.

He let out a big breath. "I'm so glad you're both okay." He shook his head and we both gazed up at the top of the slide, nearly a hundred feet up.

I took Prince's rein from Blake and stayed well back while he inched forward, a step at a time, to assess the damage to the trail. "We'll have to go bush to get around this," he said when he returned to where I stood with the horses. "It'd be dark long before we get home if we went back the way we came."

I nodded and handed him Prince's rein, then followed him and the stallion's bunched hindquarters straight up the bank beside us, leading Tessa. For nearly the next hour, we scrabbled our way up and far around the slip, finally returning to the trail just opposite where we'd been stopped.

"You all good back there?" Blake peered around Prince to check on me.

I nodded, then mounted Tessa. "I hope we don't see any more of these today." I shivered. "It's getting late."

"That's the first one I've ever seen up here." Blake frowned, then swung up onto the stallion. "Lena, the trail's wide enough for us to walk side-by-side."

I nudged the mare and she walked up beside Prince and

kept pace with him. "Good thing Tessa was paying attention, because I sure wasn't."

"You were talking with me." He winced. "Sorry, Lena. Anyway, before we were so rudely interrupted by a mere slip, you were talking about your helpful uncle," he said, with forced cheerfulness.

"Ah, yes. My uncle." I tried to smile—I could at least try to return the cheerfulness, and with the dropping temperature, after our climb, I was at least warm.

I considered for a moment. "He's convinced himself it's for my benefit, but he'd get every cent out of it, and then some. I'd have to pay it off in blood."

"It's got to be better"—Blake raised a brow—"than having no job."

"True, but I'll be putting out job applications as well.

"Of course. Where are you looking?"

"A few equine practices down east of LA and some in the Santa Ynez Valley always take a bunch of new equine track grads."

"You're determined to stay equine?"

"Yes."

"Then you should probably do it." He hesitated for a moment. "But if so, why the small animal preceptorship?"

"I wanted more experience with small animals, in case I chose a mixed animal practice after graduation, and as much surgical training as I could get. Unless you're in a big equine surgical practice, other than suturing wounds and castrations, a general equine vet wouldn't do much surgery."

"And is the practice with small animals really so bad?"

"Not really." I looked down at my hands on the reins. "Truly, it's not. It does put me out of my comfort zone, though, which probably isn't a bad thing. I understand horses' health problems so much better than I do those of small animals—it seems more intuitive to me."

"And have you been allowed to do much surgery this summer?"

"I sure have," I said with a grin so wide it stretched my whole face. "Dr. Franco's given me more opportunities than most preceptors ever get. He supervises me on surgeries a new small animal vet would rarely see, much less perform, for several years in practice." I gave him a sheepish look. "I really shouldn't complain—I'm actually quite lucky."

He nodded in agreement, and we rode on down the valley, reaching home just as the sun set.

MYRTLE STOOD WATCHING in one of the upstairs dormer windows as we walked in the gate and up the drive. I waved half-heartedly and turned back to Blake.

"She's not likely to go away tonight," he murmured. "Would you like to go out to dinner?"

"That would be lovely, but first, I don't think we could top our lunch, and second, I don't think I could eat another bite. That was truly an amazing meal. Thank you again."

"You're so welcome." His smile warmed me to the tips of my cold toes. "Let's get these horses to bed and get you inside."

After the Arabs were fed and groomed, we loitered around the barn, hanging up tack and tidying.

"It's surprisingly cold tonight, for summer." I rubbed my arms to warm them up.

"If we're not going out, maybe we could make a fire and play scrabble, or chess?"

I grinned. Chess with him would be fun. "You'd probably kick my butt if we played chess, but if we played Scrabble, Myrtle could play, too."

"Thanks for that," Blake said, with a big sigh, and he

looked straight at me, his eyes glowing. "I think it'd make all the difference to her."

"She *was* here first, after all"—I gave him a twisted grin—"and she keeps your life in one piece. That's important."

"We do, however, have more strawberries." He hesitated, his gaze locked onto mine. "Would you... like one?"

I froze, swallowed hard, and took a deep breath. "How about we eat them with Myrtle while we're playing Scrabble?"

"You're right, you know," Blake said softly, a short time later as we walked up to the house, "to keep things slow between us."

I flicked a glance up to his face, just visible in the darkening gloam.

"I have issues to work through," he murmured. "It'll take time."

I reached for his hand and squeezed it. "I'm starting to think you're everything I've ever wanted... and I'm scared, too. It'll take time for me, too." I filled my lungs and closed my eyes for a moment. "Strawberries and Scrabble? Maybe we can play chess after Myrtle goes to bed."

"You've got yourself a deal." Blake lifted my hand to his lips and pressed a kiss lightly upon my knuckles. "I've got time. All the time we need."

"You know"—I brushed the hair back out of my eyes, and my breakfast, then shook my head at myself—"Myrtle was hilarious, once she figured out I wasn't a threat."

"Three dogs and two horses can't be wrong. Myrtle's okay," Blake whispered as the sound of a door closing at her end of the house echoed up the hallway.

"Good morning, you two." Myrtle smiled. "I haven't had

such a fun evening in years." She glanced at me. "You'll give him a run for his money, I'll bet."

"I'll do my best, ma'am," I bobbed my head at her, "but I don't know if it'll be enough."

"You'll do, you'll do just fine. Can you children stay out of trouble for a whole day? I'm heading out, so be good."

"What are you up to, now?" Blake grinned at her.

"I happen to have a hot date out on the golf course with a new resident, and don't you mind which." She stuck her nose in the air and walked out front door. "And he's paying for breakfast at the clubhouse," she threw over her shoulder before it closed behind her.

"Don't do anything I wouldn't do!" Blake called after her, just before the door slammed.

My eyes met Blake's and he reached out a hand across the table. I took it and the spark tingled up my arm and warmed my heart.

"She'll probably talk him into dinner, too, just watch," I said.

"How about we ride down to the manager's office and tell them about the slip in the trail? They'll take care of it—that's why we pay exorbitant association fees."

"So, all this is managed?" I stared at him. "I've never seen anything like it."

"Think you might like to spend some time here?"

"Would I?" I took a deep breath. "Sounds like heaven."

Blake started to speak, then stopped. I waited in silence.

"Would you... would you like to stay for the rest of the summer after you're done in Santa Barbara? Maybe you could get a part-time preceptorship in Tehachapi?"

I blinked. That would take some thought.

Wasn't it a little soon to be planning life together?

He left me to my considerations for long minutes as we

neared a massive covered arena, corrals with a few horses, and a dressage arena.

"Before you make up your mind, perhaps you'd like to see the equestrian center they're developing. I'm sure you'd have some good ideas for them."

I eyed him sideways. "Now you're just trying to coerce me," I said, but I smiled to myself.

"They're making a big arena, Olympic carriage driving size."

"How did you know I've always wanted to drive?"

"Just a guess. It's always been my dream."

We meandered over the grounds and found even more arenas and some little mare motels. Most people we met stopped to say hello and chat, but we finally made it to the corporate office and told the burly manager about our find.

"Thanks for letting me know, Blake," he said. "Most people don't get that far up the northern trail. Good thing nobody was hurt."

"This good mare stopped just in time," I said, with a scratch for Tessa on the withers.

"I haven't seen a slip up there before, certainly not one that size," Blake said. "It's big—might take a while to fix. We'll definitely need access by this winter for the endurance race, though."

"Consider it done," the manager said with a smile, and shook Blakes's hand and mine. "When you get time, come down and have a look at the plans for our equestrian center. You might have some ideas to improve them. There might"— he winked at me—"even be a spot an equine vet might like to set up a little practice."

I flicked a glance at Blake, my eyes narrowed, but he shrugged and held up his hands.

"Honest, I said nothing to the man." Blake defended himself as they walked down the steps of the office. "But you've been seen here for going on two weekends now… and you know my history."

"Conspiracy, I say!" But I grinned all the same as the manager waved from his office.

"What do you say?" Blake asked when we were alone again. "When you're done in the big city, want to come up here? Ride and relax until school starts again?"

I took a deep breath, held it, then let it out slowly. "My heart says yes, but my head says no. Like I said before, I can barely feed myself and my animals on my part time wage, much less make school fees."

"I could help."

I stared at him. "You barely know me. You're certainly not responsible for feeding us." I was silent, my mind racing, then I continued. "I'm lucky Frank at ICU held my job for me while I was down south. During the summer, the full-time techs get their vacation time and we get the extra work. These summer hours, combined with my part-time hours during school, will be enough to pay my bills. And then there's my own horse, getting fat in a big pasture, and a cat to think of. I'm not being a very responsible mother to them."

Neither of us said anything for a long time.

"Maybe we could bring them down," Blake finally said, into the silence.

I gawked at him. "You're not on an airplane now, Toto. We're talking a seven- or eight-hour trailer ride. Each way, for a few weeks' visit."

"And? I travel that far to a ride."

He had a point. "But…"

"It's not a big deal."

I reached out a hand to him and he gripped it as we rode along together. "I'd love to, I seriously would, but I need the work."

"But I can—"

"No, you can't. I have to have some pride, too, Blake. Let's see how it all goes, and we can talk about this later, ok?"

"Sounds good," he said, but he didn't sound convinced. "You have to leave tonight?"

I sighed. "I probably should. I need to be at the clinic at 7:30 to open up. If anything should happen on the road over…"

"You're right. Wish I had a plane."

"You do. Planes that someone else pays for."

"True, the best kind."

"Also, I'm going to leave a little earlier today. I want to visit my mom."

He blinked. "Your mom? Where is she?"

"Mariposa. By looking at the maps, it should take me an extra hour or so to get home."

He grinned. "On a fine day with no motor homes. You never said she lived down there."

"I've been so excited about… everything." I swallowed and tried to smile guilelessly. "Guess I forgot."

"We'd best get back, then."

"We're not in that much of a hurry. What else do you want to tempt me with?"

He looked at me from the corners of his eyes. "Not so sure that's a good idea, but I can—"

"That's not"—I gave him a stern look, which cracked after a few seconds—"what I meant." I shivered at the tingles lighting up—down where I shouldn't be feeling them.

His lazy smile let me know he had a pretty good idea about my thoughts. Good thing I was heading home soon. Lord knows what might happen otherwise.

"It's good to see you, Mom," I said, and I meant it, as we clung together in the doorway of her little house in Mariposa.

"I feel like it's been years, but it's only been since Christmas," she said and wiped the tears from her eyes. "I miss you, girl."

"You did have to move all this way south. That's actually one of the reasons I took this preceptorship, so I could see you."

"You're such a darlin' girl. But where have you just come from? You've been, if I'm not mistaken, cuddling"—she picked several white hairs from my shirt—"a gray horse?" She looked askance at me.

"Yes, I went to help out at an endurance ride a few weeks ago and made some new friends. Horse friends." I beamed.

"The best kind, but come on in. Dinner's just ready. I'm so glad you're here and that you gave me *some* notice," she said, with a grin.

We got dinner on the table and sat down on her back deck. The sun, in its final throes of setting, blazed a full spectrum of purples, yellows, and oranges across the sky.

"It's beautiful," I breathed.

"One of the reasons I like it so much here. And it doesn't rain." She looked up from her fork, loaded with my favorite, lasagna. "So where have you been today?"

"Up in the mountains"—I flung one hand airily toward the east—"riding with my new endurance friends I met at the ride." I jumped into the details of the ride, treating the sick horse, and this very cool stallion I'd met.

I soon finished and jumped up to clear the table, quickly adding, "But Mom, what have you been up to?"

From the look she gave me, she knew I was hiding something, but I had good reason. Mom had been into endurance racing for years—and she still knew everyone in that world. That didn't help me much—I'm sure she'd know

Blake. After she updated me on her life, Mom looked at me, point blank.

"So, any interesting men in your life?"

I mumbled something into my crème brûlée and thankfully, she didn't push me.

She'd find out eventually, but I wasn't ready to talk about Blake. Not yet. I wanted to be sure there was something real there before I made waves. And there would be waves. After all, he was… a little older me.

Well, a lot older.

Fortunately, my mother is very patient and understanding.

My father, however, isn't. Neither patient *nor* understanding.

And that doesn't bear consideration.

11

"How was your weekend?" Ray waggled her brows at me as she grabbed a horribly burnt pot and dunked it into the sink in our apartment the next morning.

I smirked. "Not like that, but it was lovely."

"And you expect me to believe that? You two holed up together all alone in a log cabin before a fire… you *did* say something about sheepskins on the floor, didn't you?" She shook her head. "How stupid do you think I am?"

I moved her sideways and took over at the sink. "What *did* you do to that saucepan? I swear, I can't leave you alone for a weekend."

She quirked her lips. "I was outside flirting with the new neighbor and forgot it was on. I don't think he was impressed by the smoke coming from our doorway."

"I'll bet not." I shook my head. "And it wasn't like that. Sure, we like each other, but we're waiting… till we're both ready."

"For what, Christmas? Lord, girl! You're both consenting adults."

She had a point. "But this one's worth waiting for… and it

seems, when I sleep with men too soon, they drop me. I'm not willing to risk losing Blake when a little patience might make the difference."

"Hmmm… you have a point. They want it well enough, and when they get it right away, you're labeled easy. Haven't been able to figure that one out, myself."

"Me neither. That's why I'm trying something different this time. Besides…" I smirked. This would finish her. "We were properly chaperoned. He has a watchdog."

Ray stared at me, incongruous with the superman-emblazoned dishtowel she held. "A what?"

"He has a sixty-five-year-old female housemate."

It was her undoing. We laughed until we cried.

"A sixty-five-year-old roommate?" she finally got out, between giggles. "Is it his grandmother?"

"No." I was still giggling. "And not his mother, either."

"Just how old is this guy?"

"Ummm…" I couldn't tell her. She'd go nuts.

Ray stopped laughing and her eyes narrowed. And she waited.

"Well, he's… a little older."

"How little?"

I bit my lip. "A year older than my father?" I winced. "But he acts much younger… and he's a gentleman. I don't think I could find a guy my own age that's a gentleman like Blake is," I said. I sounded a bit defensive, even to my own ears.

"Can't you? What about your Dane, Jesper?"

She had me there. "Well, not one in this country."

"You obviously know Blake better than I do, but… you're twenty. He's what, forty-five? If you're as serious as it looks from here, have you considered just how old he'll be when you're fifty? When you're still bouncing around having the time of your life?"

I shook my head. I hadn't gotten that far yet. He was still

just a gentleman to me. "We'll see how it goes. Other than his age, from *here*, he's the perfect man for me. Time'll tell, Ray."

She swallowed hard and shook her head slowly. "I hope you know what you're doing."

"Me, too, but I'm sure loving it now."

Ray glanced at the kitchen clock. "And we're going to be late if we don't run now," she said, grabbed her lunch off the counter and bolted. I raced on behind her.

We were late for work.

THE WEEK FLEW by at the clinic and Fred the cat seemed happier with every passing day.

Blake called on Wednesday night. "The horses and dogs send their love, and I can't wait to meet Fred. You're bringing him up this weekend?"

I smiled, my heart warming to this man who didn't look like he was giving up on me, despite my chicken-like behavior. "If I get the go-ahead from James, I sure will. You'll need to fix him up a little room, so you can contain him and keep him in the house until his splints come off. I warn you, it'll be awhile."

"No longer than a broken leg, though."

"Yes, longer. Tendons heal slowly because there's not much room for blood vessels between the tendon fibers."

"Good to have a vet around."

"Is that the only reason you want me? Your own private vet? Isn't there a female vet already over there you can keep?" I was only half joking. I'd wondered about it before but hadn't been game to mention it.

"She's already married," he teased, but it was true. He'd told me.

I just want to be loved and wanted, truly wanted. Did he want me or just his own vet?

I nearly missed his next comment.

"It's you I want. The vet part is just the icing on a very, very nice cake."

I couldn't help smiling at that.

"And I'm starting…" I admitted, in a whisper, "to want you." At a clatter of pots from the kitchen, I wished the phone had a longer cord—like long enough to reach into my bedroom.

On Friday, I got the official word on Fred.

"He's free to go, as long as Blake brings him down next month for a checkup"—James counted off on his fingers—"takes good care that he doesn't get rubs or sores under his splint, and keeps him confined."

"I promise. I won't leave him there until I'm sure he can do all that. Besides, he has a watchdog."

He looked at me strangely, his brows nearly touching, as he headed into his first consult of the day.

I grinned at his back and returned to wrapping up a surgical pack.

"You away again tonight?" Ray bumped me with her hip as she passed.

I grinned at her and placed the pack in the autoclave, added water, cranked it shut, and pushed the red "on" button.

She twisted her lips at me. "I take it that's a yes."

"Yes."

"I was hoping you'd come out with us again." Ray's lips turned down at the corners. "You're going to be leaving soon."

"How about we go out midweek next week sometime? We don't have to stay out late."

"Sounds decadent, and good." Bouncing back, she smiled and carried on her way.

My ancient pickup seemed to be learning its way to Blake's.

"I couldn't wait to get here," I said out the open window to Blake as I pulled hard on the parking brake on Friday evening.

Blake pulled open the car door and fought the dogs off as he pulled me out of the truck and into his arms.

Though we'd only been together a handful of days, with all the midweek phone calls, (I shuddered to think what they'd cost), it felt we'd been together for ages.

"The horses missed you." He leaned back to look into my eyes, his arms still around my waist. "Especially Tessa. She much prefers you. Your hands are better, and you weigh"—he picked me up against his hard body—"definitely less than I do."

"You'd better let me down before you embarrass yourself," I murmured. "Where's your watchdog?"

"She volunteered to make dinner tonight if I went out and got a chocolate banana cream pie."

"Why is she bothering with dinner, then?" I grinned.

"That's what I asked her. Seems to think we need our veggies, so the pie's in the fridge."

I shook my head. "That's *so* wrong."

"So, you up for some riding tomorrow?"

"When wasn't I?"

"So, where's my cat?" he demanded.

"Bossy, bossy." I grinned up at him, just as an annoyed "meow" came from the cat carrier on the back seat.

"He's *beautiful*," Blake said, cuddling him close after we'd taken him out in his new laundry room kennel. Fred rubbed his head up against Blake's chest.

"Looks like he's known you for years." My heart swelled with happiness for this almost-dead cat who had a second chance at life. "Traitor," I added and rubbed him between his green eyes, where he liked it best.

"Thank you for saving him. I'm sure you did a fantastic bit of surgery." Blake gazed into my eyes and I reached up and kissed him lightly on the lips. "Did you see that, Fred?" he asked the cat. "I'll keep you around if you can make her do that more often."

I laughed and went to get some cat food.

"And so," Blake went on, shouting to make himself heard above the wind as we trotted down the trail, "I spent a lot of time on my own out running around the mountains. My mother always knew how long I'd be gone by the number of cans of mushroom soup that were gone from the pantry."

"Didn't you get lonely?" I screwed up my face.

"Nope. It was bett—I was happier that way."

"I was always a bit of a loner, too, I guess. Spent a lot of time out in the fields alone at school, hiding out. If I went far enough, they wouldn't tease me."

"About what?"

"Whatever. It didn't matter. That's where horses come in. I could be alone for hours or days, but never lonely." I smiled, remembering.

Blake grinned. "You pegged it."

We spent half of that Saturday riding, cleaning tack, and mucking stalls. That evening, we barbequed steaks and ate out on the porch while the dogs wriggled at our hips, before the big wooden rocking chairs called to us and we sat and rocked like an old Appalachian couple.

"Come here." Blake jutted out his chin at me and my face heated. His big chair had room for two and he reached out for me.

I sighed and went to him. He enveloped me in his arms and just held me... for so long, I nearly fell asleep.

"Am I boring you?" he mumbled.

"Absolutely not," I whispered, half asleep. "I can't remember feeling safe in anyone's arms in years." My heart clenched, and I stiffened, but I fought it, forcing my muscles to relax. Then I began to breathe again.

"Who was he?" Tersely.

"He?" I turned my head away.

"The man who wouldn't let you feel safe in any man's arms."

I hesitated until he gave me a little jiggle.

"He... he was a student. A few years ahead of me. Thinks he's god's gift.... but he's just a bully."

"What did he do?" Blake growled, tension locking his every muscle.

"Wined and dined, then proceeded to get demanding. When I resisted, he got rough. When I wouldn't go out with him again, he threatened me. I still have nightmares."

"What's his name?"

"It doesn't matter. He's graduated and gone. I'll never see him again."

"Did you report him?"

"What's there to report?"

"You're that scared of him, eh?"

I nodded and stared off into the distance. "It would be his word against mine. Just drop it, please. I'm happy now. I didn't think I'd let a guy near me again, but your patience won out." I looked into his eyes and his lips lowered to mine, softly, gently, in a kiss, then he lifted his head.

"Okay?"

"Better than okay. Fantastic," I said and sought his lips myself this time.

His body stiffened and hardened against me as the kiss

deepened and somehow spread between us. I opened my lips to his soft request and he asked for more. I gave it willingly and soon forgot my surroundings in the rolling wave catching us up, until a wet nose worked its way under my armpit, and I giggled.

Jake LaRue grinned into my face.

"Jake, you know just when to show up, don't you?" Blake said, shaking his head. The other two dogs crowded around, now Jake had broken the ice. We patted them and looked up to see Myrtle coming out the front door.

"We're screwed now," I whispered.

"No, we ain't," he replied.

I'd learned his mantra last week. It broke the tension when things weren't going quite to plan.

"Off again, more golf," Myrtle said, not looking down at us. "Don't wait up."

"She's getting cocky," Blake said.

Myrtle turned and shook her head. "Just leaving you two alone, or you'll never get together." She stomped off.

We stared at each other.

"Are we really taking too long?" I whispered, joking.

"Maybe. If Myrtle thinks so, we might indeed be."

"Do you think we should do something about it?"

"Got any bright ideas?" He raised a lazy brow at me.

"A few…"

"I'd like to see them… shall we go inside?"

My heart pounding, I slid to the deck and stood, reaching a hand out to him. He took it and rose, then kissed my hand, picked me up and carried me over the threshold and up the stairs.

WE DIDN'T AWAKEN until the dawn peeked through the east-facing windows and spread its light over Blake's big four-poster log bed.

"Good morning," he whispered, his arms snug around me.

"Mmmm… I don't think they get any better," I said and rolled over, still in his arms, to face him.

"No, surely they don't. And it's only Sunday morning. We have another whole day more." He took my lips with his and pulled me hard against him.

"But what about the horses?" I leaned back and looked into his hooded eyes. Eyes that were anything but sleepy.

"Found a note slipped under the door an hour ago. Myrtle's feeding everyone. Complete with threats." He held it up and read it aloud. *"If you come down those stairs before ten, I'll murder you both."*

"I'd sure hate to see her get arrested for a double murder," I murmured.

"Me too. See? She even brought up a breakfast tray."

I shook my head and chuckled under my breath. "Wonderful woman."

"After you, the best," he said. He sat up and twisted sideways to reach his bedside table and my mouth dropped open at the ragged white scar zig-zagging its way across his back. I shut it hastily as he returned to face me, a bright red berry from the plate between his fingers. "Now about those strawberries…" he whispered. "I seem to remember…"

I forced my attention away from my vet student mind's automatic classification of "the severity of a wound required to leave a defect of that size"—the *pain*—and onto his gaze, hot and molten above me. His eyes gripped me in their sway as he lowered the berry to my lips and I bit into it, my insides once again pulsing fit to burst. He put the rest of that delectable bit of sweetness into his own mouth. After that, fruit became the last thing on my mind for quite some time.

After I managed to forget the horror of the ridged pale mark that jagged its way across his torso.

"About time, you two," Myrtle barked, when we finally stumbled down the stairs later that morning.

Blake frowned. "But you told us not to get—"

"About time you got *together*." She grinned like the cat who ate the cream. "I had to take things in hand, but you've finally done gotten on with it."

"Truth be told," I said to Myrtle, with a twist of my lips, "we didn't want to shock you."

She shook her head. "Girlie, when you've been around as long as I have, you learn not to waste love when it's offered. You never know when you might not have the chance anymore." A shadow passed over her face, then it was gone. "I'm off," she said.

"Another golf date?" Blake's brows shot up.

"So many men, so little time. They'll just have to take their turns. And today, I'm putting them all off to play golf with the girls," she said as she slammed the door.

Sunday passed in a sleepy haze. The horses even obliged, their paces slow and relaxed. I stayed Sunday night, barely able to drag myself from the warm bed before the dawn's first light.

"You drive safely, you hear?" Blake said, concern in his voice. "You're not too sleepy?"

"No," I smiled. "I'm fine. I'll talk with you tonight, eh?"

"Promise. I'll ring after I land in Bakersfield."

He leaned in my window for one last kiss.

"Bye, bye." I waved and headed back to the coast.

12

"The phone!" Ray dashed up the last few steps and scrabbled for the apartment keys in her purse while balancing two big bags of groceries on her hip.

Like a tag-team member, I raced after her and dropped my bags on the deck, then fished in her bag until I hooked the recalcitrant keys and opened the door. Ray followed up by trotting into the living room, abandoning her bags on the sofa, and reaching for the phone.

"For you," she called from the living room. When I reached her, she covered the mouthpiece. "It's a man," she hissed. She wiggled her eyebrows and headed into the kitchen.

"Hi darlin'." Blake's voice coated my heart with chocolate with just words.

"Hello there, yourself," I said, my voice melting, along with the rest of my body.

"Just wanted to hear your voice. Got home okay?"

"Sure did. *And* made it to work on time."

"So what are you doing on Wednesday night?"

"What's Wednesday?"

"A certain favorite girl of mine's birthday."

"Oh!" I blinked. "I'd forgotten. Probably nothing, since it totally slipped my mind."

He laughed. "Well, I wanted to say 'Happy Birthday' for tomorrow. I hope your day is special. I just landed in Bakersfield and wanted to call before I headed home."

"Thank you… for thinking of me… and for another lovely weekend," I whispered, as a fist curled pleasurably down deep in my abdomen.

"There'll be many more, I hope. Well, bye for now, and have a great birthday tomorrow," Blake said. "Sleep well."

"THAT WAS"—I wiped the sweat from my brow with the back of my wrist after my last surgery on Wednesday—"particularly nasty." I surveyed the surgery room. It looked like a battle scene, with blood drying sticky over drapes, instruments, and me. The metallic smell of the blood still tingled at the sides of my tongue.

Ray shuddered. "It would have been nice if we'd seen all those fractures on the x-rays."

I sighed. "Sometimes they don't displace enough to see them on the films right away. Without a few days of bone resorption to show us the fracture lines, I guess that's just the way it is."

"Lucky we had a K-E apparatus to fit him." Ray picked up a few of the clamps and half-pins, plus the two stabilizing bars we hadn't used, scrubbed them, and dropped them into the ultrasonic instrument cleaner. "We'd never have been able to stick together all the fragments we screwed and plated without it.

"Lena, someone here for you," said the receptionist, as she opened the door.

In walked a man hidden behind the biggest bunch of long-stemmed roses I'd ever seen. "Ms. Lena Scott?" he asked.

"Yes?" I stared, searching for his face behind the blooms.

"Delivery for you. Please sign here."

"Let me take those." Ray reached for the crystal vase containing the stems so the flower man could hand over his clipboard. He fumbled for a moment and nearly dropped the vase before Ray could grab it. "That vase nearly went into our purses," she said with a laugh.

"I can't believe this," I breathed, and scrawled my signature. "Thank you."

"Have a nice day." He nodded, spun, and disappeared.

"Wow, just wow." Ray handed the bunch to me and my heart swelled so much I could barely breathe. I fossicked amongst the thornless stems but couldn't see a card. "No card, but no matter. There's only one man who'd send roses like this." My smile was so wide, I thought my face would split.

Ray leaned over and inhaled their scent. "Mmmmm... yep, that man's a keeper, all right. A keeper." She beamed over her shoulder and went back to scrubbing the blood off the remaining instruments.

I was still beaming an hour later, just on quitting time.

"We haven't planned anything for your birthday." Ray frowned. "Would you like to go out?"

"Really, after the afternoon we've just had, a bath and crashing on the sofa sounds good, but let's see how it goes."

"You've got me there." Ray smiled. "I didn't want you to feel neglected on your special day."

"Not a chance of that." I chuckled. "Not a chance."

BLAKE OPENED the door of the veterinary hospital and the

bells hanging on their cord jangled, stilled, then rang madly again as the door clicked shut.

"May I help you?" The redheaded receptionist gave him a sunny smile.

"Yes please, I'm here to see Lena."

"Do you have an appointment?"

"No. She doesn't know I'm coming." He moved closer to the front counter. "In case you don't know, it's her birthday."

"And you must be….."

"Blake. I don't want to disturb her, but do you know what time she's finishing tonight?"

"Should be soon. More flowers?" She beamed at me. "She's a lucky girl. Come on back, I'll take you through. She's straight through here."

Lena saw him in the doorway and took three steps toward him, beaming, then her eyes dropped to the flowers in his hands. She stopped like she'd been shot and her mouth dropped open.

"Tell me you're not allergic to lilies?" Blake raised a brow at her and handed her the flowers with a smile. "Happy Birthday, darling."

Lena smiled and accepted the flowers, cradling them as if they were a baby, then gave him a big hug around the flowers. "No, I love lilies, thank you so much. They're beautiful, and even my favorite colors." Her voice quivered, and she almost looked embarrassed for a moment. "And you're *here*!"

"Couldn't miss my favorite girl's birthday!"

"Hello," Ray said, and introduced herself. "Lena is too awestruck to remember."

"Sorry, Ray," Lena said, and bit her lips together.

"Nice to meet you. I've heard all about you," Blake said, as Lena stepped back and reached down into a cupboard for a vase.

"Likewise." Ray laughed.

"I've come to take you out to dinner, Lena, if you wish. I came early so I didn't miss you, but don't let me get in the way. I'll just sit out in the waiting room—"

"You can sit in here. We're almost done."

"Are you sure?" He frowned.

"No problem," said Ray. "We should be about ten minutes. We'll just finish up the kennels, then we'll be right out." She stuffed a handful of magazines into his hands. "Here's some reading material for you."

"Nice clinic," he said as Ray walked away. It'd been built from an old house, modified to feature the best of the old as well as the new. Maybe they could use some of these ideas in Lena's new clinic at Elk Valley—if it all worked out between them. He glanced around the treatment room, taking note of the deep tub under the treatment table, the lab in the corner, and the flowers—

The flowers.

Not only flowers, but nearly two dozen long-stemmed, thornless blood-red roses.

"More flowers…"

He shuddered and forced himself to walk over to the blooms.

His heart constricted in his chest when he found the florist label. They were for Lena, all right, but no card. A surreptitious glance around the room revealed no little pink or white card.

Maybe they were from her father.

Yeah right, Sagan. How smart are you?

He tried to breathe deeply to keep his vision clear.

Lena is nothing like Jana.

His ex-wife had never looked at him like Lena already did.

Or had she?

He swallowed hard and tightened his jaw. With a glance at

the lilies, he picked up a National Geographic and forced himself to turn the pages, one after the other.

This wouldn't alter his plans for tonight.

Lena was worth keeping.

I RACED after Ray into the kennels, flung the door closed, and pillowed my head on my forearms against the back of the closed portal… as if that would keep Blake from seeing the roses. "Oh my god. What just happened?" I whispered.

"We need to find that card," Ray murmured, with a shiver.

"I have *no* idea who sent those roses… and they're in there with Blake," I hissed.

"You must have *some* idea. No man you haven't told me about?"

An uncomfortable niggle raced up my spine. *Tim?*

"There was a guy I was going out with, but it wasn't serious. I've only spoken with him once since I came south. Just before the endurance ride."

Ray winced. "Your father perhaps?"

I winced right back. "He's overseas, in the middle of nowhere. No phone, probably not even a telegraph. And he certainly wouldn't have sent roses."

We stared at each other.

"We need to find that card," we both said at the same time.

"Let's get done here. We've got a man waiting," Ray said.

My chest tightened further, but there was nothing we could do now.

Fifteen minutes later, the three of us walked out the back door of the clinic and climbed the stairs to Ray's apartment.

"I'm Ray's roommate while I'm in Santa Barbara." I smiled

up at Blake. "We can get changed here. How fancy are we getting?"

"As dressy as you want. We're going to *Le Chez Soir*."

Ray inhaled sharply. "Lena, we'll raid my closet, okay? You didn't bring anything *remotely* suitable for *Le Chez*."

"'One's Own Backyard', and it's that dressy?" I blinked.

"Trust me. I've been there once. You know which forks to use at a place like that?"

I nodded. "Sure do. Mom taught me to survive anywhere, from a big international dinner to the hippie house next door." I looked up at Blake with a smile. "I won't embarrass you. Promise."

"I'm not worried about that." He kissed me lightly on the lips. "We're paying them to serve us dinner. Our manners are the least of their concerns."

"I like the way you think," I said.

This evening would be fine. Maybe he hadn't even seen the flowers.

Men didn't tend to notice things like that.

Did they?

THE FEW REMAINING pieces of *Le Chez Soir's* sterling cutlery and the silver Victorian under-plates glittered in the light of the million-faceted crystal chandelier. I sat back. My tummy was too full for the sequined, strapless black gown I'd borrowed, and I wasn't at all sure how I was going to teeter back to the truck along the waterfront's brick walkway on Ray's six-inch heels.

"Happy Twenty-First Birthday, Lena." Blake lifted his champagne glass to me once again. "Enjoying your dinner and the restaurant?"

I smiled at the gentleman seated across from me. Blake

looked comfortable in his tux and it suited him. "Yes, though I don't think I want to make a habit of it. I haven't seen such opulence since my grandfather's passing several years ago."

"I'm sorry." Blake frowned. "I didn't mean to remind you of sad times."

"It's okay. He lived a full life—more than a full life." My fingertips caressed the ridges of the fine gadroon borders on my under-plate, so like those in my grandparents' home and their Scandinavian fine furniture import stores. "He packed more into his life than most men ever dream of. Did you know he finished the Tevis nine times?"

Blake blinked. "You mentioned he'd done it several times, but you didn't say how *many*-several. That's nearly a record."

"I think that was one of his only regrets." I twisted the narrow stem of my champagne flute in my fingers. "He didn't earn his 1000-mile buckle."

"If he's anything like you, I'll bet he gave it a good shot."

"He did, and his wife, a lovely Swiss woman, rode the Tevis as well. I have a wonderful photo of her climbing Cougar Rock on her gray Arab."

"I'd like to see that sometime." Blake's voice was warm, his eyes dark in the candlelight as he reached a hand across the table to take mine.

"I'm sure you will." I smiled at him and glanced around the room. "This reminds me of the World Trade Club, my grandfather's club and *the* businessman's club in San Francisco. It's in the Ferry Building on the waterfront, much like this." I looked out the window at the glittering Pacific Ocean."

"I've never been there."

"It's lovely. It has wood-paneled walls and floor to ceiling glass sliding doors opening out to balconies over the water, and they carve a new ice sculpture every night for the buffet centerpiece. The last one I saw was my favorite—a magnificent dolphin playing in the waves."

He shook his head. "Sounds wonderful."

"It was pretty exclusive—and personalized." I couldn't help smiling. "The *maître d'* always remembered to bring out my grandfather's burnt toast when dinner rolls were served."

He laughed.

"Thank you, Blake. This is an amazing birthday surprise. Dinner was exquisite."

"Would *mademoiselle* like dessert and coffee?" Our waiter appeared out of thin air, the napkin folded over his arm as snowy and crisp as the shirt beneath his dinner jacket.

I looked across at Blake. "You go ahead. I'm too full, but thank you."

"I'm done, too. Prince'll toss me if I eat any more." He glanced up at the waiter. "No, thank you, but our compliments to the chef."

"I will convey that to Chef. Thank you very much."

I excused myself to go to the ladies and teetered back afterwards. I'm not sure if the champagne helped the shoes or hindered them.

"The men are watching you," he remarked.

I quirked a brow at him. "It's the dress."

"It's what's *in* the dress." His eyes glimmered in the shadowy room.

I glanced around at the men. Some turned their heads away, but others glared at Blake with hostility. I shook my head. "They do seem to be watching, but they're frowning at you."

"They're just jealous. How many men my age have a gorgeous twenty-one-year-old on their arm?" he said, but his smile melted just a little after that.

BLAKE GAZED around *Le Chez Soir*, quelling the sideways looks of the other male diners with just his eyes.

Lena smiled, but she bit her lip and turned her gaze away, out over the bay. The men had looked on indulgently while he and his date had dined.

The man and his daughter.

Once he and Lena finished their dinner and moved closer to each other, holding hands, they'd seen the truth.

What the hell.

She was mature, bright, lovely, and fun. And he was only twenty-five years older than her. Heck, she was older than his son... *maybe.*

A shiver ran up his spine.

It'll be okay.

He took a deep breath and glanced across at her, glad the smile had returned to her face. He wanted to see her happy forever. "Lena?"

She met his eyes, one eyebrow raised.

"Would you like to take a turn on the balcony with me?"

"My mother warned me about men like you," she smirked, "but, yes, please."

Under the moon, the ocean was a glittering sea of stars as he took her hand and kneeled before her.

Lena looked at him strangely, then her mouth dropped open.

"Lena, would you do me the honor of becoming my wife?"

She stared, swallowed hard, and thought for a moment.

Blake's heart was in his throat as she began to speak.

"We've known each other for such a short time, but... I think we were made for each other." She bit her lips together for a moment, took a deep breath, and gave him the answer he wanted. "Yes, Blake, yes. I will marry you."

He leapt to his feet and took her face in his hands. The kiss was sweet and lasted forever.

13

"I'm sorry I have to leave so early," Blake said the next morning, craning his neck to watch as I struggled to button his pilot's four-bar gold epaulette into place for the first time.

"You came all the way down here to take me out for my birthday, midweek." I smiled and smoothed my hands down his brilliant-white pilot shirt. "And you even asked me to marry you. Who am I to complain?"

He laughed and kissed me atop the head as I buttoned the second epaulette into place. "So now that you can feel more secure about school for the next two years, you'll stay down here the rest of the summer?"

I stared up at him in silence, a thousand thoughts racing through my head.

He looked sideways at me. "What?"

I took a deep breath. "I still have a life up north, Blake… animals, a house, and a job I've promised to return to. I can't drop everything, just like that." I snapped my fingers. "Can you give me a little time to get used to the idea? You've had time to think about it, but it's all new to me."

"But you don't *need* to work this summer, or during the rest of school, for that matter. That's the whole point. That's why I asked you to marry me now."

"The other point"—I tried to keep my voice steady—"is that every day in my ICU job, I'm practicing to become a better vet. I wouldn't get that opportunity as a student, even as an equine track student."

Blake glanced at his watch and his jaw tensed. "I've got to go, but can we talk about it this weekend? You're coming up?"

"Of course"—I smiled at him—"I'll be there Friday night."

"I'm sorry, but I've got to run. I'm flying jump-seat and they won't wait. There's money on the table for a taxi back home."

"Thanks again for last night, and this morning, and…" My face heated, and he smiled. "I'm glad I'm going to be your wife. We'll make a good team. Fly safe, my love."

"Don't let the little dogs bite. Love you."

We shared a quick kiss, then he ran down the hallway for the waiting taxi.

I locked the door and let myself fall back onto the bed for a few minutes, gazing around the lovely honeymoon suite Blake had reserved for us, shaking my head. This man was well on his way to spoiling me for anyone else, ever.

I finally rose and stepped out the French doors onto the balcony overlooking the ocean. This sort of luxury hadn't been in my life for many, many years, if ever.

The student life just didn't quite compare.

"Ahhh… that feels good." I smiled at Blake as I sank backwards onto the sofa in his log-lined living room, late the following Saturday afternoon. I'd managed to drag myself into the shower after slithering from Tessa's saddle half an hour ago. And we'd only trotted for four hours up hill and down dale.

"And you want to ride a fifty-miler?" Blake raised a brow at me. "Sure you're fit enough?" He chuckled.

"I assume I'll have ridden a bit more regularly to condition myself," I shot back, and laughed. "But I promised to help you with the new dog bed. Let's get to it."

"Don't you sound excited." Sarcasm. He opened a bottle of juice and poured a glass for each of us.

I roused myself and sat with him at the kitchen counter. "Blake." I looked him squarely in the eyes. "It's my last weekend here, and I promised I'd help."

"You *promised* to discuss that. The part about it being your last weekend here." His words were steel-tipped.

"True. You know I'd love to stay and ride, play with horses, and you, of course," I added, trying for a smile, "but it's impossible right now. I've asked my house-sitter if he can stay on longer, but he's committed elsewhere, and I can't just dump my animals."

"We can go get them."

"Blake, I have work that I need to do to live, and it's part of my education. Don't you want me to be the best vet, ever?" I wrapped my arms around him, wheedling now.

He gave me a look, something between a twisted grin and a frown. "But..." He let out a big breath. "I wanted you to feel secure, that you're loved, and that you didn't need to worry about money."

I bit my lip. "I appreciate all of that, but there are, and always will be, some things I need to do for myself. It doesn't mean I love you any less."

Blake was silent for long minutes. "What if your uncle succeeds in talking you into working at his place? That's a pretty good offer," he added grudgingly.

"Yours is better. All of yours. And you." I reached my

fingers up to slide through his hair and brought his lips close to mine. "I'm not going anywhere away from you, if that's what you're worried about. All of this"—I waved my hand around the house, encompassing him, the dogs, and the horses out the window—"has all made my uncle's actions so much more clear. He never really believed I'd get into veterinary school in the first place. Wouldn't surprise me if he figures I won't graduate. I have little to no interest in a broodmare or racetrack practice. I worked at a track awhile, and that world isn't for me." I couldn't help an involuntary shudder.

Blake kissed me then, and the peck deepened into a driving desire. I clung to him.

"Just because I'm not staying down here doesn't mean I don't want you, Blake," I murmured, on the verge of tears. My voice sounded deep and throaty to my ears. His eyes darkened as he held me hard against him, then picked me up and headed for the stairway to a place we could let our tensions out in a more constructive way than fighting.

A long time later, Blake slowly sat up. He moved to the window, where he stood for long minutes, just staring out over the valley. When he turned back, his face was ashen.

"What is it?"

"Nothing. I'll just miss you."

I reached for him and he slid into bed beside me. "I will return, and I will marry you. Just see me through the rest of my school, will you? Please?"

He nodded and held me close. My fingers ran over the scar and he flinched. I swallowed hard. He'd never mentioned it and I hadn't had the guts to ask. It was time.

"What happened?"

He was silent so long, I thought he hadn't heard me. Finally, he spoke.

"One of my mother's men friends."

I pulled myself away so I could focus on his eyes. "Your mother's what?"

"She had a steady stream of men—most of them drunks. They didn't appreciate a boy in the way. This one used a piece of firewood to see I stayed away."

"Didn't your mother do—"

"She didn't care enough to stop it and I learned to love mushroom soup from a can, out in the woods on my own. No one hurt me out there. I'd rather not discuss it further."

I clung to him like a limpet. "Thank you for telling me," I mumbled into his chest.

"You're the first I've ever told," he whispered.

"Maybe it'll help. You couldn't have done anything to deserve that, you know."

"Just drop it."

I swallowed hard and was still. We held each other for what felt like hours before he rolled away and reached a hand up to wipe the hair from my face.

"Thank you. Just for being you," he said.

"I'm not so good at being anyone else." I was silent for a moment, then, "Blake?"

"Mmm?"

"Can I ask you a question?"

He nodded, turning a wary look upon me.

"What happened to your previous marriage?"

Blake was silent for a long time, then he looked away. "We grew apart, I guess."

I wasn't fooled. Something had happened, and I can't imagine it was good.

He held me tightly and then looked me in the eye. "You hungry?" he asked.

I nodded.

"I thought after we feed the horses, we'd go get a bite from down the road."

I gazed around and out the window at the peaceful valley, devoid of restaurants. "Down the road? Where?"

He smiled. "There's a charity dinner tonight at the clubhouse and I thought you might enjoy it. Dinner and dancing."

"You had me at the dinner, but the dancing'll get me there for sure."

"A LOVELY DINNER, THAT." I sighed and patted my belly, gazing around the golf club reception hall, which had been converted for the evening into an impromptu dining room. "Thank you, Blake. I'm so glad I brought over my little black dress."

He arched one elegant brow. "So am I. You're always gorgeous, but"—he reached his fingers toward my long braid hanging over one shoulder and tugged it lightly—"you're particularly lovely tonight."

A man dressed in black passed by our table and headed for a table covered in black boxes near the stage.

"A DJ, even?"

He grinned. "I already put in a list of requests. Do you have any?"

"Whatever he plays will be just fine. Do you dance?"

"Only a little."

That made me smile. Some of the best western swing, Latin, and ballroom dancers I've ever met told me those same words.

And yes, as we started, he showed me just how "little" he could dance. Waltz, foxtrot, quickstep and western swing, to be exact.

"Yes," he admitted, when I cornered him after the first few

sets. "I've done a bit of dancing. Two step?" He nodded at the floor.

"Thought you'd never ask," I said with a laugh. " 'A little', you say... more like, you probably competed."

"Only a little," he conceded.

"As a vet school class, our only vice is dancing. My classmates Dane and Toni and I knew how to dance western swing before vet school and we taught the rest of them."

He was silent for a moment, a shadow passing over his face. "And where do you dance?"

"Usually at *The Classroom*, a bar with a big dance floor, lights, you know the sort of place. We go as a group, so it's not a pickup situation." I smiled up into his face.

But he didn't return it. "I wouldn't think you'd have time to dance," he said tersely.

I raised my eyebrows at him. "We usually don't. But when you're studying twenty-four-seven the rest of the time, a couple hours a week could be considered allowable?" I ended on a question, with a hint of a challenge.

He took a deep breath and spun me along the line, around and around, as he two-stepped behind me. When we reached the end of the dance floor, he spun me to a dizzy halt as the music ended, then placed a hand on the small of my back to guide me, wobbling a bit on my high-heeled cowboy boots, to my seat.

"Drink?"

"I'll just have water, thanks. I only have one drink when I'm dancing."

He nodded and disappeared, returning with two waters and a better attitude.

What was that about?

I bit my lip and looked across at him, staring off into space. He was usually so happy and positive... but I was starting to realize there were still many things I didn't know about this man.

And I'd just promised to marry him?

I hoped the darker ones wouldn't amount to much.

I MUST HAVE IMAGINED the shadows on his face last night, because this morning, there was no room for darkness in the bright spark that was Blake as he whirled me around the kitchen in his log house before breakfast.

We finished that dog bed, my normally bossy self probably irritating him more than a bit, and took the horses for a—slightly shorter—ride.

"I'm going to miss you terribly, Blake," I said, for the umpteenth time, as I shoved Prince's supper hay between the rubber straps of his hay barrel. The horse was a Houdini for dragging his hay out and strewing it over the gritty ground, perfect conditions to wind up with sand colic.

"Not half as much as I'll miss you," he returned, "but you'll be too busy to miss me. I'll keep myself occupied with getting two horses ready for us to compete in January. You *do* want to race Tessa, don't you?"

"Wouldn't miss it for the world," I said with a smile. "I'll get as much riding in as possible and start running again. Wouldn't want to embarrass you or Miss Tessa."

"You could never embarrass me half as well as I do myself."

"Un-likely," I said, and bit my lip. "I have to go pack. My mom's expecting me for dinner, and it's the last time I'll be able to see her before I go north."

He gave me a twisted smile and took my hand to lead me back to the house.

We packed my bag and he grabbed the snack he'd put

together for me from its place on the kitchen counter, and together we walked out into the cooling evening air.

"I'm going to miss you," I said again, "and this place." He kissed me, then opened the passenger side door.

"Oh hell," I growled, as my purse tipped out into the gravel. "It must've been sitting against the door." I shook my head and ducked down to gather it all up. "I really shouldn't pack everything but the kitchen sink into a bag designed for a wallet."

"Sorry, I should have looked before I opened the door."

"Not your fault." I smiled and returned to picking everything up, knocking the dust off, and shoving it back into its place.

A pink card lay half-covered with gravel. I frowned and shook it off.

Blake looked up. "What's that?"

"I don't know. Never seen it before."

"It's a florist card." He pointed at the logo. "FTS"

I turned it over.

Happy Birthday, Lena! Miss you! Can't wait to go back to Kirkwood again, this time in the summer. See you when you get back, Jeff

14

I blinked and stared at the pink bit of trouble in my hand. "Oh my god. *That's* who sent the roses. You remember the roses at the clin..." my voice trailed off at the look on Blake's face.

"I remember the roses." His voice could have cut steel.

"I thought... I thought they were from you. There was no card."

"Clearly, there *was* a card. You're holding it."

"But I never saw it," I whispered as my heart squeezed in a vise. "It must have fallen into my purse. Truly, I never saw it before this moment," I managed as tears filled my eyes.

"Who is Jeff?" He spat each word.

"A guy... just some guy I was going out with... but it wasn't anything serious."

"Red roses? Were you sleeping with him?"

"Sometimes, but..." I stopped, searching for words, then straightened up and clamped my jaw tight before I went on. "Blake, he means nothing to me. He was a friend. Sometimes we had sex. It was casual. We weren't ever together in the way you and I are. I told you I'd marry you—that means you'll be the last man in my life. That's what marriage means."

"Not to everyone."

"Well, it does to me," I growled. "When I give my word, it stands. Period. If you don't trust me, tell me now and you won't see me again."

Blake closed his eyes, his lips moving silently. When he opened them, he reached for me. "I'm sorry. Trust doesn't come easy for me. I didn't learn it when I was a child and my ex-wife certainly didn't help me learn it, either. I swore I'd never trust anyone again, and then, look what happened?" He gave me a watery smile, then pulled me hard against him. "I want to, but it's… hard."

I took a deep breath, trying to let go of my anger. I'd never given anyone cause to distrust me and resented my word being questioned… but, and it was a *big* but, he had his reasons. I needed to have some patience with him…

I'm blessed sure he'll need patience to deal with me plenty of times in the future. This is just paying it forward.

"Honestly, Blake, about the card, neither Ray nor I ever saw it. When you came to the clinic"—I bit my lips together and gave him a little smile—"we were desperate to find out, after you brought flowers, too. When you walked in, I was about to thank you for the roses."

"That's what the hesitation was." He tried for a smile, too.

I nodded and squeezed him around the middle. "That's what it was. I had no idea who they were from. Can we agree to trust each other?" I said in a small voice.

He nodded and held on tighter.

Our upcoming separation by distance stretched out in my mind clear to eternity.

It was bound to be a long, long wait, but it'd be worth it.

MOM'S SMILE stretched from ear to ear as I parked my old truck before her house. I really needed to tell her tonight—this was the last time I'd see her before I headed north next weekend.

I managed to delay until we'd nearly finished the peach cobbler.

"So what's his name?" Mom said, out of the blue.

"Who?" I played dumb, fingering my fork.

"The guy you don't want to tell me about." She smiled and reached out a hand to pat my arm. "This is a long way from Santa Barbara, so there must be some real interest. Is he a nice boy?"

Silence. "I don't think you'd call him a boy… more of a *man*."

I hadn't cared about Blake's age, but I had an idea Mom would. I had no plans to even *tell* dad, who was a year younger than Blake. I can't imagine him understanding.

"'Man'," Mom tried again. "Did you meet him at school?"

"Nooooo…" It was now or never. I took a deep breath. "We met at an endurance ride," I said, as brightly as I could manage.

"Oh? Nice! What's his name?"

I gulped audibly, cursing myself for my cowardice. "It's Blake Sagan."

"Blake… Sagan." She tilted her head, her brows narrowed over a little smile. "Nice family. I know them from our endurance years. But surely, you mean his son, Jordan."

I cocked a brow at her. "No, Mom. Blake."

She blanched, then swallowed hard. "If it's the same man I'm thinking of, isn't he a little old for you?"

I took a deep breath and tried to get my heartbeat to slow a little. "We don't think so and we've been having the most wonderful time. I'm *so* over the guys my age. I'm tired of being hurt."

She blinked. "And you think an older man won't hurt you? How do you figure that?"

"Well, he's a gentleman."

She waited.

"He doesn't try to get into your pants at the slightest provocation. I spent three weekends up at his house before he even—" I broke off, my face burning.

Mom closed her eyes and gripped the table edge before her. "Have you thought just how old he'll be when you're—"

"Yes, Mom," I interrupted. "I've thought of all that." I think I might have growled that last bit.

"How does he feel about your new career as a veterinarian?"

This one, I could handle. I smiled and breathed again. "He's excited at the idea of having his own vet." I laughed.

She considered for a moment. "Yes, I can see he'd be happy for that... and how will he feel about his young wife out at all hours working on horses for young, virile men as he gets older and older?"

I blinked.

"One last thing... have you thought about children?"

"Children? I'm only twenty-one, Mom!"

"And if you decide to have them, just how old will he be then? And when the children are teenagers?" She was silent for long moments. "I'm not asking you for answers, darling"—she took my hand—"but I want you to consider these questions... before it's a done deal. If your mother doesn't ask them, no one will."

I gulped and gripped her fingers until my knuckles turned white. "I love you, Mom, but he's really very special."

"I know he is. He's a wonderful man. You'd like Blake's son Jordan, too, and he's just your age. All I ask is that you go into it with your eyes open."

I got up and went around the table to hug her. I was lucky to have her, even if she wasn't saying what I wanted to hear.

I didn't have the heart to tell her about the engagement. Time enough for that later.

A lot later.

"Engaged?" Ray gaped like a fish out of water.

"Well?" I raised both brows at her.

"But you barely *know* the man! And, have you thought about what I sa—"

That wasn't the response I expected and my face heated as I struggled for words. "Of course, I—"

"Lena," the receptionist interrupted from the doorway, "there's a dog in the exam room for you to see. Here's the record. Go ahead and check it out. The doctor will be in soon."

"Thank you," I said as I took the file and tossed a look over my shoulder at Ray.

The spaniel's people were pleased the rash on their pet's tummy was probably just a response to fleas and the hot, steamy weather we'd been having. They trotted out the door with their flea control and some medication to sooth the itch, waving as they left.

Ray was waiting for me in the kennels, eyebrows lowered and her lips a hard, firm line.

I took a deep breath and looked at her.

"So you've said yes? Where's the ring?"

"We'll worry about that later."

"What's his rush?"

"He'd hoped…" I winced and tried again. "He had in mind to support me… because then I'd no longer have to work… and he hoped I'd change my mind and stay down south with him for the rest of the summer."

Ray looked at me sideways, her forehead furrowed.

"I told him I had to go back to work and continue learning at my ICU job."

"And…"

"He wasn't impressed, but he got over it… *I think*."

"Do you really? How many men that age do you know? How many that have a woman in the work force, with an actual *career*?"

I was stunned. Something I hadn't remotely considered.

Ray took a deep breath and seemed to give up. "Well, anyway, it's your last week here," she said, grumpily, "so we're going to have some fun before you go."

I tried to smile, but I'm not sure I made it. Our ideas of fun didn't always coincide, but I'd do a lot for my friend. As she said, it was my last week.

"Oh, and Ray," I swallowed hard, "I, or we… found the card."

"The car—oh! So there *was* one?"

I closed my eyes, unable to speak.

"That bad, was it?"

I just nodded. "That bad."

Ray put an arm around my shoulders and sat me down on a shipping crate. "I want to hear all about it," she said.

AFTER I DROVE home to Northern California and played with my animals, my next stop was the vet school. I headed for the ICU office, and was pleased to see Frank, our hunk of an ICU supervisor.

"Lena," he said, in his most wheedling tone, "can you work full time for the next month until school starts?"

"Full time, I don't know… what hours?" I said casually, just to wind him up.

His brows narrowed, and his mustache twitched. "I thought you wanted—"

"I'm just having you on, Frank. Of course, I'll work." I laughed. My friend Jess had already told me he was scrambling desperately to cover shifts. "Gotcha." I gave him my cheekiest grin.

"Brat." He shook his head. "Thanks."

"In case you hadn't heard, I just got engaged. Blake wanted me to stay down south with him until school starts, but I told him I had to return to work, so I'd best make good use of my time."

"Engaged, like, to be *married*?"

"Yes, that kind, and pick your jaw up off the floor, Frank." I laughed. "I'm not *that* bad a catch."

Although he was the worst flirt in the world, and a good dive buddy to boot, he managed to evade even the most ardent and beautiful pursuer. I don't know how he did it.

He shook his head. "Better you than me."

"I think Blake would agree," I said, with a chuckle. "When do you need me?" I pulled out my calendar and proceeded to fill it with dates.

"How's your horse doing?" he asked when we were done.

"Fat, bored, and happy to be out on the hills. I thought of letting him stay there for the rest of the summer, but I'd miss the riding and need to get fit for an endurance race later in the year."

"Which race?" he asked, and I told him all about Prince, Tessa, Blake, and the Elk Valley Springs 50.

"Hello, darling," Blake said when I picked up the phone

that evening. "How was your day? Glad you got that long drive out of the way yesterday."

"Hello yourself," I said. "It was good. I start work again tomorrow."

"In ICU?"

"Yes. Frank needs me."

"Frank? Who's Frank?" He almost, but not quite, growled.

"He's my boss, remember? Yes, he's handsome, and yes, he's a friend. No, I'm not sleeping with him and never have. Any more questions?" I was only half-joking.

"It's okay. I get it." He laughed a little. "So how's that horse of yours? Did your cat miss you?"

"Horse is good, but I think the horse and cat would rather I stayed away. The cat's probably gained two pounds and has been spoiled to death. She now disdains cat food."

"Oh no." He laughed. The tension broke, and I could breathe again.

"Did you get to work the horses today?"

We spoke of his animals until it was time to get off. He told me Fred was being a good cat and goodbyed me with a kiss in my ear.

I sat, looking around my little old house until my eyes fell upon the stack of board exam study notes I'd begun compiling. With a sigh, I pulled the top one onto my lap, opened it, and began to read.

This would be my life for the next few years: eat, study, clinical rotations, work, and if there was time, sleep.

WHEN I GOT home after working the next night, or the wee hours of the following morning, to be exact, there were five messages from Blake on my answerphone. Their tones became more testy as the call times progressed.

"Hello?" came the groggy voice on Blake's end.

"Hi, sorry it's so late, I just got home from work."

He was silent for a moment. "Where have you been? I've been worried about you."

I blinked. "I've just got home from work."

"In the middle of the night?"

"Yes. ICU runs 24/7. Right now, I'm on swing shift, four to midnight, so I'll be home at this time for most of the week."

"Ah, okay. Well, I'm glad you're home." He still sounded grumpy.

"It'll be a bit tough to talk, other than early mornings before you leave for work. I won't be home this week until one a.m., if not later."

"Okay. Sorry I growled. I miss you already. I'm not sure how I'm going to do this, but I will."

"Good night. I'm shattered," I said, still more than a little put out.

"Goodnight, sweetie," he said, and hung up.

I was well-awake now, so I went to bed with my study notes on my lap to make the most of the time until I felt like I could get to sleep. Another morning coming up with a book on my face and the light still on. My nose must be flattened from all the books that landed on it during my college years.

I ARRIVED HOME the next day in a howling summer gale to find a message from Ray. I called the clinic to talk with her at lunchtime.

"How's it going up there?" she wanted to know.

"It's great up here, but I don't think Blake's very happy. Our work hours aren't coinciding, so we'll talk this weekend."

"That's tough. Everything is fine down here, we miss you.

Just a mo—" A muffled conversation, then, "Hey Lena, I have to go. A patient just came in."

"Okay, great to talk. Give my love to all."

I was just a little bit lonely after that. Empty, even, as thunder shook the little house. The lightning came soon after… too soon. I glanced outside to see how the horse was taking it. He had a full hay net and didn't seem to care. He only cared when we were out riding in it. I smiled, thinking of our last exciting stormy ride.

A car revved its way up the gravel road to my little farmhouse and turned my gaze that way.

And closed my eyes, leaning my head against the window, heart going a mile a minute. Now was not a good time.

A broad smile on his cherry visage, Jeff hopped out of his fancy blue car. It was different from the fancy red car he had last year.

I swallowed hard and went to the door. I tried to smile as I opened it.

"Well hello, Lena. Missed you something awful," he said and gave me a hug. His arms still around me, he leaned back and looked into my face. "You okay?"

I nodded slowly and he let his arms drop from my stiff body.

"So, did you have a good summer? I just got back." He reached for my hand and began to drag me toward his car. "Come on and see my new wheels"—he glanced up at the roiling gray clouds—"before it pours. We can take her to Kirkwood before school starts."

I tried to breathe while he rattled off the specs of his new blue car. I missed the whole thing. Not a huge surprise. If it didn't have four hooves and a mane, it simply didn't compute.

"Lena?" He stopped and turned me around to face him. "What is the matter? Where's my girl? Have you lost her in Santa Barbara?"

I didn't have the faintest idea what to say. Had I?

"Ummm… thank you for the roses." I frowned, but gave in to a giggle. "They dropped me into dog poo, though."

"You're welcome." Jeff smiled. "I thought you'd enjoy them, all on your own down south."

"That's just it. I have a boyfriend now," I blurted out.

"Oh."

I peeked up to see him looking down at his feet, disappointment lining his face. My heart twinged in my chest.

"What's the matter, now?" I said, giving him a little shake. "It's not like we were ever together so this isn't splitting up, or anything. He's a *real* boyfriend."

He blinked. "Like, a real, *real* boyfriend?"

"Like a real, *real* boyfriend."

"A forever one?" He didn't seem to be getting it. He'd never wanted commitment in the entire time I'd known him.

"A forever one," I said, with a laugh.

"I didn't think… like…"

"What? Don't you think I could get someone who actually wanted to stay with me, not just sex?" I said, probably more hotly than I'd meant.

He chewed the inside of his cheek then straightened up and looked me in the eyes. "And how exactly did my beautiful, I imagine they were beautiful, roses dump you in the proverbial?"

I closed my eyes and finally opened them, looking at him from beneath my brows. "The card must've fallen out of the bouquet, into my purse, so I didn't know who sent them…" My face was steaming. "I nearly thanked Blake for them… then nearly died when he carried in his own bunch of flowers."

"Oh no…" He was shaking his head, his lips pressed into a tight line holding back the laugh.

"And we found your card a month later… as I was driving

out to head home. It wasn't"—I quirked my lips—"my finest hour. He's a little jealous." Now it was my turn to bite my lip.

"I won't apologize for sending flowers, because I'd still send them tomorrow," he said flatly.

I winced. "Hopefully without the Kirkwood reference."

"Are you going to invite me in?"

"Of course." I smiled and led the way. I got him a drink while he sat down on the sofa.

"So where did you find this Casanova?"

"We met at an endurance ride."

"Makes perfect sense, for you," he said, then fell silent. The only horsepower he liked had wheels, not legs.

"He's a pilot," I added. "He has lovely horses and he built his own log cabin. A big one."

Jeff pursed his lips, his brows touching. "That's a lot to do by the time you're thirty."

"Did I say he was thirty?" I blinked. "He's older than that. More like his forties."

"Forties? Isn't that a bit old for you?"

"Some men mature like a fine wine," I said tightly.

"By the time you get to his age, your fine wine'll be getting a bit vinegary," he said, with a twist of his lips. And he didn't look like he was joking.

"Why Jeff, I do believe you're jealous!" I shook my head. "You never wanted more than a casual sexual thing. You made that clear long ago," I said with a frown.

He looked away as I stared at the side of his face.

"I knew you were busy with school and couldn't commit, so I never… asked." He finished on a whisper just before the thunder and lightning hit simultaneously and the skies opened up so loudly we couldn't hear each other talk for a full minute.

I looked outside to see rain already overflowing the gutters, then turned back to him in time to see him looking at me with sad puppy dog eyes, which he wiped with the back of one hand.

"Don't do this. Not now, Jeff."

He shook his head and stood to go as my own eyes teared up. I'd wanted him to care for me, too, for a long time, but he'd made it clear… It was too late now. Simply too late.

I asked him about his car and stood to get him a wet cloth. Talking about his cars always cheered him up.

He sat up and scrubbed at his face, talked for awhile, then soon stood to leave. In the doorway, he bit his lips together for a moment.

"Thank you again for the roses," I said, "and thanks for stopping by."

"Look, Lena, I'm sorry I don't get the chance to really be together with you, but I'm… glad you have someone to love." He touched my hands with his, and shot out the door into the storm while I watched the rain drip down the windows. The blue car turned and disappeared down the drive the way it'd come.

My imagination ran away with me, as it does. Things that would never be.

Even the house was crying.

It was a long week. Blake and I didn't manage to talk much that week, between his leaving at five for Bakersfield to fly out and my getting in at one. Our talks were short, at best.

"How about we just talk on Saturday?" he said one morning when he'd just woken me up to talk at 4:45 a.m.

"Sounds like a good idea," I slurred. I'm not sure what else I said, but I think I fell asleep while he was still talking.

15

"So, how's Lena getting on back up north?" Myrtle looked at Blake, one brow raised.

He twisted his mouth and said nothing for a moment.

"I haven't heard you talking on the phone for days."

"Yeah, well, she's never there," he said, with a scowl.

"Is she out partying?"

"No." Blake squirmed. "She's working. And studying. And lord knows what else, but she's on swing shift and we can't manage to talk." Myrtle knew just how to trip him up from a good pity party, and he had an idea what she was about to say.

"Well, boyo, that's to be expected. She already has a life up there. I'm sure she'll fit you in as best she can."

"I know that, but…"

"No buts about it," she said, with a frown. "That girl's been working more than hard for most of her life to get where she is right now. Cut her some slack," she said, and she stomped off.

Great. Another pushy woman. Just what I—

He cut off his thought and tightened his jaw. She'd done

nothing wrong and he was just going to make himself, and her, miserable.

Good job, doofus.

He made himself a sandwich and headed out for a ride. At least he had that.

SCHOOL STARTED AGAIN, and rather than getting easier, everything got that much harder. Clinic rotations started early, with treatments to be done before rounds with their rotation service clinician, then depending upon your service, treatments, surgery, seeing patients and clients, or running around barns all day. And always the incessant records—S.O.A.P.s, surgical records, anesthetic records, treatment records, and research and preparation for rounds presentations. And then there were sometimes still classes.

Yes, this was what I came to vet school for, but I'm being buried alive here.

There were lonely animals at home, and training for the upcoming endurance ride. I fit in a run whenever I could, most days.

And then there was Blake.

Meant for each other or not, there was not much left of me to give.

He came up on the occasional weekend, and we trained together—in the few minutes I could spare. He worked on his pilot updates while I studied.

"You know?" he said with a wry grin one Sunday as he pulled the last of his outdated airstrip maps out of their binder and replaced it with the current one, "I've never been as current in my updates as I am now. I have so much time while you study. There's got to be a plus here." He put his book down and came over to my desk. "Are you ready for a break? You've been at it for three hours."

I blinked and set my pen down, then rubbed my eyes. "I have so much to do, I can't stop, but I can't do any more, either."

"Let's go out for some dinner. I'll feed while you get a shower."

I smiled my thanks and stumbled off the bathroom.

When I emerged from the shower, I felt almost human. And ravenous.

Blake came in the door just as I finished dressing. "Better now?" he asked and hugged me.

"Yes, and dinner sounds fantastic. We need some time to ourselves, from"—I took a deep breath—"somewhere."

"Let's go," he said, and held the door.

"Would you like to drive?"

He reached out a hand for my keys and handed me into the passenger seat. "Sure. You need a break."

"I wish I could find more time to spend with you when you're here on the weekends," I said. The guilt was getting to me.

"The time's just not there," he said as he buckled his seatbelt. "I don't like it, but short of you quitting school, there's not much you can change, other than stopping work."

I gritted my teeth. "You know why I won't quit."

"Just sayin'." He stuck the keys in the ignition and held up his hands. "As I said before, I can support you."

"I don't feel right about it."

"Don't you trust me?"

"Don't you trust *me*?" I flung back at him. I didn't have enough patience for much right now, and certainly not this.

He sighed and clamped both hands on the steering wheel.

I closed my eyes and held my peace until we got to the

restaurant, then I tried again. "I've been training as much as I can fit in."

"That's good," he said, automatically. "I'm busting myself every moment I'm home to get two horses ready to race."

I swallowed. "I'm not sure what I'm going to do about the animals over Christmas. My usual house-sitters will all be away. I might have to bring them down with me. That should create chaos with yours."

"We'll do whatever we have to." Short.

"Look this isn't getting us anywhere." I covered my face with my hands. "I'm sorry, I'm being terrible, but I'm past exhausted. Can we just eat and go home, then cuddle till we fall asleep?"

I looked up to see his gaze softening, the hard lines melting a little. He reached for my hands and I gripped them for dear life. "I just need some rest," I whispered.

"We both do," he said. "We both truly do."

That night, he held me wrapped tight in his arms until we dragged ourselves from bed and I dropped him at the airport at five a.m. the next morning to fly to Bakersfield—to work, and home.

BLAKE PICKED up the phone one Sunday morning, a month later, to hear Lena's voice.

"Hello?"

"Well hello there, busy girl. Missed you yesterday. What did you get up to?"

"Worked a shift and a half, came home and fell asleep. Sorry I didn't ring."

"That's okay."

"Whatcha' doing?" The wistful sound in her voice tugged at his heart.

"Well"—he paused—"sitting on the porch in the morning sunshine with Fred and the dogs."

She was silent for a moment. "Don't you have anything better to do? Stuff to learn?" Her voice raised a bit.

He blinked and took a deep breath, considering, while trying to be understanding… instead of simply snapping at her. "I'm sure I do, but… isn't it okay to enjoy life a little?" You were fine sitting here on the porch with me when you were here."

"I just… " She fell silent. "I'm sort of… stressed, but that's no excuse, really."

"If you'd seen the things I have, darlin', you'd understand."

She didn't answer.

"I know you're tired. You're burning the candle at both ends. I am too, getting Prince and Tessa fit, working, and worrying about you. No small feat for either of us."

"I guess so," Lena said, and she sniffled, then began to cry.

"It's okay, sweetie. God, I wish I were there to hold you."

"But then I wouldn't have time," she wailed. "I don't have time, I push you away, you cling, and I feel trapped.

"And then, and then," she sobbed, "my stupid uncle is pressing me for a decision, and a loan… now he wants me to finance it. Whether I tell him 'no, thank you', or 'go to hell', the whole family is going to go ballistic. I don't know what to dooooo…" her cry broke off and stopped. All he could hear is her breathing and the occasional sniffle.

"Look, Lena, I'm coming up this weekend. I want to see you and talk. We're going nowhere like this. Is it okay?"

Silence.

"Is it okay?"

"Sorry, I was nodding 'yes', and of course, you couldn't see me. Yes, I'd love to hold you. But do you have time?"

"No, but I don't think we can wait."

"Me either," she whispered.

"I love you," he murmured. "Can you get something to eat and go to sleep?"

"Yes, I will."

"Now?"

"Okay. Love you. Bye."

The phone clicked dead and he sat there for long minutes, staring at it.

He couldn't go through what he had with Jana.

And she was even younger.

He wouldn't.

But if he didn't let himself trust anyone again, he'd be as lonely as he had the past six years… and most of the rest of his life.

And that didn't bear thinking about.

AT A KNOCK, I opened up my front door to Blake's concerned visage. "Oh Blake!" I cried, and lunged into his arms.

"Whoa, whoa, girl. Are you okay?"

I shook my head. "Everything's too much."

"Well, we'll do what we can to help that this weekend, okay?" Blake picked me up like I weighed no more than a child and carried me to my big old overstuffed chair. He set me in his lap and held me while I sobbed, his fingers stroking my hair until I quieted.

"Well, what's first?" Blake said, after I'd run out of tears.

"Eat, probably," I mumbled.

"When was the last time you ate a decent meal?"

"Mmmm… not sure."

"Well, that's first, then."

We were fine until halfway through Sunday.

"Lena," Blake said, "you said something the other day on the phone. It was the only thing that really stuck, and I have to say it worried me."

I stared at him.

"You said you felt trapped. I don't want anyone to feel trapped by me."

I was silent for long moments, then finally managed to whisper, "When you cling or get jealous, or make snarky comments if I tell you I've done something with someone else, male or female, I think you don't trust me…"

He gulped. "I trust… I trust you."

"I don't think so," I said, my voice becoming stronger, "and I wonder"—I hesitated for what felt like a lifetime—"if it'll always be like this. I tried, when we were down at your place, to let you know you could trust me, that I'd be there for you, but it seems like… when we're apart, that trust disappears. That's what jealousy means to me. That you don't trust me. And I can't, no—I *won't* live with that." I finished on a whisper.

He took a deep breath and let it out slowly.

"And it makes me wonder…" I said, "what really happened in your marriage."

"That was nothing like us."

I looked hard at him. "Are you so sure?"

"Of course," he growled.

"Okay…" I still couldn't believe it, but that was his story. I'd accept it, for now.

"What else do we need to air?" he asked, and gritted his teeth, his jaw as tense as the rest of him.

"Other than your serious prep for the big fifty-miler coming up, I don't see you wanting to go anywhere with your life. You work, and you're 'gettin' by'. Is that all you want from life? I mean, you're just happy to sit on your deck and look at the view. Is that important?"

He stared at me. "I fly jets. Do I have to keep striving for something? Just because you chose to become a veterinarian and kill yourself for eight years of straight-A study, does that mean I'm a lazy so-and-so? I used to tease you about your intensity and serious pursuit of your dreams and goals, but other than school, your flightiness and unpredictability remind me more and more of Jana—" he broke off.

"Jana." I swallowed hard.

"My ex-wife," he finally bit out.

I waited for him to tell me about it, but it looked like it wasn't going to happen. I reached a hand out to him, but he didn't even look at it. He wasn't done.

"More *importantly*, have you ever had experiences that let you see what life is really about? Strive and strive, so you can fly men, in the hundreds, home in body bags? Boys going to R & R with bleeding stumps of arms and legs? Young men... *young* men, in the thousands, who'll never see the light of day again? Don't talk to me about what's important, if you don't think celebrating *life* is."

I froze. "What?"

He looked away, his face like stone. "Nothing," he finally muttered, and began to walk away.

"It's important," I whispered as I grabbed his jacket, chastised. "Please tell me about it?"

"Never mind," he growled. "You could never possibly understand. Just leave it"

I closed my eyes—unable to look at the pain in his—my fingers still gripping denim, and then our arms were around each other.

"I knew you struggled with self-doubt," he continued on, "and so I encouraged you to go past it, knowing I'd probably lose you when you had more confidence. It terrifies me. I don't think I can do it… again." He finished on a whisper and I clung harder. "It makes me want to clutch you to me and never let go."

"And it makes me feel," I whispered, "like I'm drowning."

"What are we going to do about it all?" he said.

"I don't know, just hold me, Blake, just hold me, please. I don't know if I deserve you, but I'll try to understand."

"I will, too," he said, into her hair.

I BEGAN my small animal rotation the day after my argument with Blake. I was determined to enjoy my time upstairs in the small animal clinic, although it was away from the beloved horses I understood so well.

After only a few days of scrambling to learn the systems up there, I ended up with a nasty respiratory infection. The stress of school and our relationship must have wiped out my immune system completely.

"I haven't had one like this in years," I told Blake on the phone, then had to hold the phone away from my ear as I hacked, my lungs rattling. "When I try to run, I can't do anything but gasp for air and my eyes are streaming all the time."

"Lena, you've got to stop. What did the doctor say?"

"Doctor?"

"You know, that person you go to when you're sick? Sort of like a veterinarian for people. Come on, Lena." He finished on a growl.

"I don't have time to sit in Student Health."

"You're sick. Go tomorrow, please. Promise me?"

"Okay," I croaked, then coughed my lungs out again.

"Look, I'm getting off the phone so you don't keep talking. Take some cold meds and get to bed."

"I don't have time. I have to study for rounds in the morning. In rounds every morning, Dr. Sing looks at me and starts spitting questions at me full speed while he frowns at me like I'm an idiot, and I break into tears."

"Oh, Lena."

"It's got to get better. Maybe if I study even more, I'll have the confidence to stand up to him. I've heard he thinks people who go equine track are too narrow… he probably"—I broke off, with more coughing—"thinks he's broadening my horizons."

"Lena, go to bed, now. Please," Blake begged. "And go to the doctor tomorrow, or I'll have to come up there and drag you in. I don't have time, but I'll make it."

The doctor at Student Health didn't take long.

"Severe allergy to cat dander," he said, with a wince, knowing I was a vet student.

"Thank god I'm equine track," I whispered. "I knew I was allergic to cats, but it's never been like this—only sniffles and congestion."

"Be thankful for small favors," he said, with a smile. "You're twitching, though, Lena. I know what med and vet school are like. You look awfully stressed, and it won't help your immune system."

I tried to take a deep breath and coughed some more. "Yes," I squeaked.

"Try this inhaler," he said as he pulled a box out of a drawer in his desk. He opened the container and showed me how to use the plastic and metal contraption.

I breathed in the medicine, coughed a few times, then did it again. As my hand containing the inhaler lowered to my lap, I took one tentative breath, and then another, and I stared at him. I closed my eyes and just sucked air in and out of my lungs for a minute, smiling. It was like magic. I could breathe again… and I didn't cough at all.

He grinned. "Like magic, eh?"

My mouth dropped open, and I breathed again. I nodded. "Thank you," was all I could say.

"Some anti-allergy tabs should help, as well." He grinned widely as he scrawled a prescription on a white pad. "Try them and let me know how it goes. And see what you can do about the stress levels, eh?"

I thanked him profusely and headed back to the teaching hospital. It was good I'd gotten the breathing problem sorted, because the news there was all bad.

16

"I made it to the doctor," I told Blake that night on the phone.

"I knew you could do it. You sound better." He sounded so pleased, I could hear his smile through the line.

"The inhaler works like magic, but..." I swallowed hard, not sure how to say this. Failing wasn't in my vocabulary. "Unfortunately," I barely managed at a whisper, "it's too late for the rotation."

"What does that mean?"

"It means my small animal medicine clinician, Dr. Sing, has decided I'm not mentally up to it, due to my performance of falling apart in response to his grilling in rounds, and he has failed me for the rotation." I finished on a sob.

"Lena, Lena. Hold on. What does that mean?"

I couldn't breathe, my chest was so tight.

I couldn't say the words.

"I don't know," I hedged, "I've been called into the Dean's office… tomorrow."

"I'm sure it'll be all right," he said, his voice soft.

I gulped. "It won't be all right. It means… it means… I won't be able to graduate on time."

There was a stunned silence on the other end of the phone. I had some idea what might be racing through his mind… and it wasn't going to be all right. Not now. Not ever.

"It'll be okay," Blake whispered. "Call me as soon as you know, okay? Do you want me to come up?"

"No, it…" I struggled for words. "I wish I had some cherry pie," I blurted.

Silence.

"Pardon?" Blake said.

"Cherry pie." My voice was stronger. "But they're out of season."

"What, in heaven's name, does cherry pie have to do with anything?"

"Mom used to make it for me when I wanted to die," I sobbed.

He made comforting noises. "I love you. Now… can you try to get some sleep, please? I realize I sound like a broken record."

After a deep breath, I agreed, and we hung up.

Tomorrow would be a test.

I DON'T KNOW how I made it to the dean's office. I'd thought I was a mess before, but by the time I got there, I might have been a murky puddle, for all the sense I could make of my brain.

"The dean will see you now," the secretary said with a smile that I suspect was meant to put me at ease.

I mumbled something to convey gratitude and stumbled through the door she held open for me. Right in front of me sat the frightening man himself.

Pull yourself together.

I was only *in* this mess because I couldn't handle my emotions when a man snapped at me. I'd best buck up or turn around and walk away from the dream I'd held close for as long as I could remember. I filled my lungs and forced my jaw to tighten.

"Miss Scott?" He raised a brow at me.

I nodded and flicked a glance at the Class of 1988 photo on the desk before him. He knew it was me. Just a formality before he...

"Would you like to sit down?" He indicated the comfy chair across from him.

As I sank into its leather-bound depths, I knew why he'd offered. The chair was like a cuddle, and it warmed my heart so much I was able to smile at him. "Thank you," I murmured. "Please call me Lena."

"Lena, then." He smiled. "I understand you had some difficulty in your Small Animal Medicine rotation."

I swallowed hard and nodded.

"Would you care to tell me your thoughts on the situation?"

"I'm sure Dr. Sing has told you everything."

He raised a brow at me. "He has. However, I'd appreciate your thoughts on the matter. You're nearly a full-fledged veterinar—"

How could he be so cruel? So close, and now he was going to rip it away?

My lungs didn't seem to belong to me and I gasped for breath for a few moments before I remembered my inhaler. I whipped it out and sucked on its plastic nozzle. After a moment, I was composed again, my jaw clenched tight.

"Are you okay?" His brows nearly touched. At my nod, he continued. "As I was saying, you're nearly a full-fledged veterinarian. What, and I'm sure there are many, are the extenuating circumstances I need to know, from your viewpoint?"

I stared at him for a moment.

I was going to get a chance?

I straightened my spine. "Well, sir, within a few days of starting the service, I came down with a serious respiratory complaint. A rattling, croup-like cough and draining sinuses which seemed to progress to bronchitis. When I finally went to Student Health, I was diagnosed with severe allergy… to cats." I winced at the dean. "That didn't help. I understand the medicine of cats and dogs, though that of horses comes more easily to me, so I put a lot of extra time into researching and working up my cases. I'm sure my sleep suffered. I was trying my very hardest and it seemed Dr. Sing was determined to push me to, or past, the edge. I became terrified even thinking about his rounds. After awhile, all Dr. Sing had to do was look at me with his frightening frown for the tears to start, but when he derided me or snapped at me, it was all over.

"I realize vets have to deal with all sorts of people, but this is the first person in this entire school, or in any of my previous schools, with whom I have had such a problem. I'm an ICU tech and work with clinicians and owners day and night. Never a problem. I don't know what else to say." I gazed into his eyes as I bit my lips together. I forced my fingers to release their grip on the side of my Pierre Cardin suit skirt. The wool would never be quite the same again.

"Well, Lena, I can understand your problems. I'm glad you've sorted out your allergy, and for your sake, I'm glad you want to become an equine vet." He smiled at me. "However, Dr. Sing is an experienced clinician and if he's concerned about your ability to perform as one of our graduates, I can only bow to his decision."

Tears welled, but I *would not cry.*

"It would mean you may not be on track to graduate on

time and could potentially be required to repeat a year. However"—he looked directly at me, his visage rigid in the face of impending tears—"if you can find a clinician or resident in the Small Animal Medicine Service who would be willing to take you on during a break, you'd have another chance to prove yourself."

My mouth dropped open as my mind raced. I hastily slapped it shut and struggled to think. "So you mean," I hesitated, getting my head around it, "I could still graduate?"

He smiled and shook his head. "Your record here, from your previous clinicians and teachers, is exemplary, as is your work in ICU. Small Animal Medicine is a major rotation, but I'm sure you'll do fine in a makeup rotation."

I jumped from the seat and reached across to shake the dean's hand. I wanted to hug him, but that seemed a bit farfetched, so I left it. "So I just have to find a clinician to take me during Christmas?"

"That's right." He added in an aside. "I happen to know an excellent resident from New Zealand who might be shorthanded over that time and could use another pair of willing hands. He's a very thoughtful and kind man, as well."

Ah, that would be Brant.

I smiled. The dean had pegged him. If I had to describe the Kiwi, I'd have used the same words. With the weight of the world sliding off my shoulders, I thanked the dean again and ran to the teaching hospital, and Brant.

"I'm so glad you can repeat the rotation and complete your course this year, honey," Blake said. He couldn't tell her how relieved he was. She wouldn't have to wait an extra year and this hell they were living through would be over.

"Me, too. Thanks so much for your support."

"So when can you repeat it?"

Lena sighed. "I'm so happy. I can make it up right away. Over Christmas, if the resident he mentioned will have me."

"How long is the rotation?" Shards of ice began cutting into Blake's chest.

"It's three weeks. I should be able to start as soon as school is out."

Now Blake's heart froze solid in his chest. "That's through Christmas… and the ride."

Not a sound came through the phone.

"Lena?"

"I'm here," she whispered.

"What is it?"

"I was so relieved, I… I forgot."

Blake bit his lips together. He wouldn't, he *couldn't*, say the things screaming to get out.

"Blake? Talk to me?" Lena said on a sob, her voice sharp with fear.

"We'll just have to make it work, won't we?" he said, between clenched teeth.

"I guess we will," she murmured. "I should be able to talk with the resident shortly. Brant wasn't there when I stopped in earlier. I'll see what we can work out."

"You do that."

"I have to leave for work, but I love you."

"Love you too. Goodnight."

Blake sank into a seat at the table. His thoughts spun in ever-widening circles. Finally, after what seemed an eternity, his gaze snapped to the coffee mug sitting in front of him. The veterinary school mug Lena had given to him.

Would it ever end?

He'd had enough. He picked up the mug and flung it with all his strength at the solid oak door. Score: Door-one, Mug-zero. He scowled. It should have helped, but it didn't.

"What the hell?" Myrtle shouted from the top of the stairs.

"Nothing," Blake growled, starting to feel a little bad.

"What are you doing, Blake?" Myrtle eyed him sideways when she saw the shards of pottery from the foot of the stairs.

He ignored her, his head in his hands.

"How long have you been sitting there?" demanded Myrtle.

He shrugged.

She clattered around the kitchen for awhile while he contemplated his fingers against the tabletop.

"Tell me," Myrtle said, as she plunked two mugs of steaming hot cocoa on the table. "I'm listening."

I LOOKED up from the record I was writing in the ICU office. Surgery residents Kit and Robert, along with the anesthesia resident Sarah Morton, faced the ICU stall, where a black Thoroughbred stood, its belly wrapped in rolls and rolls of Elastoplast over its abdominal suture line. They'd performed colic surgery on it last night.

"Lena"—Kit turned to me—"do you have this horse's record?"

I nodded and stood to hand it to him as he came into the office.

"Thanks," he said. "The referring vet will be here soon, and I suspect he'll be in a right snit if anything's not perfect. I remember him as a student."

I'd only been listening with half an ear while I searched for some equipment in the back of a cupboard. I shut the door with a frown and turned to the clinicians. "Kit, can you possibly keep an eye on him for a moment? He keeps trying to rub out his catheter so I need to find some sort of a cradle for him. It's sutured in, but mere suture is no match for this boy, and tape's not cutting it, either." I smiled at him as my face heated. He was something else. I don't know how they pick the residents—they all have exceptional CVs, that goes without saying, but somehow they manage to find the most gorgeous men and women for our surgery and medicine services.

"No problem, we'll be here for the next fifteen minutes."

"Great, thanks," I said, and slipped out the back door, heading for the storeroom.

Behind me, Robert's Texan drawl echoed through my head. "He ought to be here soon. He called the front desk fifteen minutes ago and gave the girls at the desk a hard time. We'll have to talk with him about that."

"You have some idea it might make any difference? We're too close in age to him—not official enough. Thank god he's moving to Southern California."

"Now if we could get Dr. Rye in here," Kit said, "he'd listen to him, but mere residents like us? Or a woman? Not a chance in hell."

"He doesn't like women, eh?" Sarah said. "What did you say his name was?"

"Barnett-Payne," Robert muttered. "And he doesn't like much of anybody. Be sure it's reciprocated."

I stopped like I'd been shot and didn't wait to hear more. I bolted to the storeroom and locked myself in. Thank god there was a phone in here to call the front office. "Mary? Could you please page Frank for me and ask him to meet me in the storeroom?"

"The ICU storeroom?"

"Yes, thanks."

"No problem," her sweet voice said, and she hung up.

I froze at a knock on the door and sat in silence in the darkness, behind a shelf for good measure.

"Lena, are you in there?" Frank asked. At the sound of jangling keys I ran to the door and opened it before he could even get one into the lock.

I stood behind the door while he came in.

"What the hell? What are you doing in here in the dark?"

I shut the door and locked it, then turned on the light. "Thanks for coming, Frank," I managed, my voice and the rest of me shaking, "but I need your help."

"Are you okay?" Frank's brows narrowed.

"Can I swap anyone anywhere else in the barns to work for the afternoon?"

He stared at me. "What's the matter?"

"You know that colic in ICU?"

"The black Thoroughbred?"

I shuddered. "The horse is not the problem, but the referring vet is."

"Who is it?"

"Remember a student from last year, Gareth Barnett-Payne?"

He winced. "Sure. Hard to forget."

"Well, he's here."

"And you want to be out of ICU, why?"

"We have a history... a scary one." I swallowed hard.

"Very scary, by the looks of it. Are you sure you don't want to go home?"

"No, but if I can stay out of the way, I can still work."

He took a deep breath. "I don't like seeing you like this, but if you want to stay, they can use you over in B-Bar. Go ask Betty to come on over here."

I shook my head. "Thanks. I'm sorry to do this to you."

"No problem," he said, and patted me on the back. "I'll keep an eye out for him, and you."

I went the long way around and found Betty. She was

happy to go into ICU and she was tough. If anyone could stand up to the jerk, it was her.

I kept my head down and worked hard for the next hour.

"Arggghh!" Betty growled, as she walked up to the stall I was working in. "What a jerk!"

"Who?" I asked.

"That jerk of a referring vet on the colic horse in ICU. Thinks he can push me around—and the residents, too. I don't know who the hell he thinks he is, but he's a real special case. He had Janette in tears after five minutes of perusing the horse's record. That's when Dr. Rye showed up—right in the middle of it all. He kicked him out, while the cretin groveled and brown-nosed him and Dr. Salisbury."

I swallowed hard. "He has respect for somebody?"

"Only the top-level senior professors."

"So glad he's gone," she threw over her shoulder, as she continued on her way to get some meds from the pharmacy.

I took a deep breath and glanced around, my heart constricting in my chest as I realized he could be… anywhere. One hand in the pocket of my scrubs, I fingered my blunt-blunt bandage scissors and an extra pair of sharp-sharps that had found their way into my hand as I scrabbled around in the storeroom.

I turned back to the little appaloosa in the stall beside me. "How did you"—I capped her catheter off and proceeded to untwist the hopelessly tangled mess—"manage this?"

She gave me a nudge and rubbed her head against my side. I couldn't help but chuckle at her, thankful she'd allayed my terror for a few moments, anyway.

"Little ratbag. I think you did this on purpose to get some attention. You're far to well to be here," I said, and kissed her spotty nose.

She would have done justice to a fine bit of Celtic knot work, but I finally managed to untangle the IV lines, reconnect the catheter and get the life-giving fluids going again.

I gave the appy a final pat and stepped backwards out of her stall, looking once again over her drip set, then reached for the latch. Two hands gripped my shoulders.

17

Heart in my throat, I spun and jerked away from my attacker, then froze, my sharp-sharps against his abdomen just beneath his ribs—staring in horror. It wasn't Gareth at all, but my boss.

Frank stared right back and didn't move a muscle. "Oh my god, Lena! You're that scared of him?" He gently took my hand with the scissors and moved it out of the way, then wrapped his arms around me.

We'd been friends for a long time and I basically collapsed against him, muttering something that even I couldn't begin to decipher.

"I came to tell you he's gone, and that you didn't need to worry. He's *persona non-grata* here for awhile."

I managed to fill my lungs and my brain started to work again. "Thank you, Frank," I murmured, and lifted my head. "I'm sorry"—I nodded at his tearstained shirt—"and I almost stabbed you."

"Having a little experience with the guy, I'd have understood. You were *involved* with him?"

"He's good at hiding it. Or used to be."

"Glad you're away from him, then. Look, it's a little early, but you head on home now. Someone's there?"

"Nope."

"Well then, head on over to my place. Leslie will be there by now. You can have dinner with us. I'll ring her."

I put everything I had left into the smile I gave him. "Thanks, Frank. I owe you one."

"You owe me nothing. Just stay away from him."

"You've got that promise. Forever would be too short a time. I'm off."

"BLAKE!" I whipped open the door of my little house and flung my arms around him. "I wondered why you wouldn't answer the phone. I thought something had happened." I couldn't stop the tears that rolled down my cheeks.

"What are the tears for?"

"I'm glad you're here," I said, and kissed him.

"I'm surprised to find you at home," Blake said, his voice tight. "I couldn't find you this afternoon or tonight when I landed, so I got a jump-seat to Sacramento and just came up." His jaw was twitching.

"I had a terrible day," I said, with a shudder.

"Mine hasn't been so great, either."

"Come on in, I'm so glad you came. How did you know I needed you tonight?"

He held me at arms length and really looked at me then, his eyes narrowing. "You've been crying."

I'd washed the tears off my face, but doubtless I was still blotchy from bawling with Leslie on their sofa until Frank came home.

I nodded and told him the whole sordid mess.

As the story progressed, his demeanor changed from

annoyance to anxiety, and on to pulsing anger with Gareth. I'm not sure which worried me more, but it was good to be held all night.

So good.

"And so," Lena told Blake the next morning, "Brant, the Small Animal Medicine resident said if I start my rotation as soon as school finishes and work through the shorthanded Christmas time, I can finish a little early. Frank will let me off for my ICU shifts, and I could come home a few days after Christmas and have a week before the ride."

"That must have taken some work to figure it out." Blake was still annoyed with the whole thing, but just hearing it was exhausting. Lena *was* trying her best.

"So I'm sorry, but I'll miss Christmas." Her brow wrinkled and she worried at her lip. "At least I can get the animals taken care of, since it'll be after Christmas," she said, hope in her voice.

"*Grrrrr...* I'm so frustrated, but if *I'm* frustrated, I can't imagine how you feel," Blake said. "I'm sorry, Lena. I just want us to be together."

"I do, too."

"So," Blake took a deep breath, "have you and your classmates been doing any dancing?"

She pulled back and stared at him, her face rigid. "Seriously?"

"You said you all did it to blow off steam."

"Yeah, well, these days I need to hold on to all the steam I can, and we're all scattered to kingdom come."

He couldn't help feeling comforted at that. The thought of Lena dancing with other men... no matter how innocent... it just didn't improve his attitude. "What do you have going on tomorrow?"

"Work and study," she said, automatically. "It's Sunday."

"Can I take you out to breakfast?"

She inhaled and let it out slowly. "I have a study group in town at eight and start work at four. Can we do lunch?"

"Is that all the time I get? Lunch?"

Lena closed her eyes for a moment. "Look, you didn't tell me you were coming up. Don't get me wrong, I'm glad you're here, but I'd have made different plans if I'd known."

"When you *do* know ahead of time, you're still too busy. Face it, you don't have time for me," Blake growled.

"I don't have time to breathe or sleep, much less do fun things. I have ridden my horse *twice* since I got home. *Twice*." Lena's eyes blazed.

"You were so upset, I couldn't just let you deal with all this on your own," Blake snapped. "What do you think I am?"

"I don't know!" Lena yelled. "You know I don't have any time, you show up and get mad at me for not making more of it! If I knew how to make more time, I wouldn't be such a nutcase." She slumped to the sofa, head in her hands.

Blake sat down on the coffee table, just in front of her knees, and reached out for her hands. She was limp. "Lena," he whispered, "Lena, look at me."

"I'm too tired to even open my eyes," she murmured.

"I'm sorry. I know we're both exhausted. It's late. Let's go to bed."

She nodded, but didn't move.

Blake picked her up and placed her carefully in bed, tugged her clothes off and then his own. She was asleep even before he pulled her close and curled himself around her.

"So how are you doing, Lena?" Blake's voice crackled over the line.

"I'm missing my mom. She's back east and with the hours I'm keeping, I can't get hold of her when she's awake, either."

"She'll be back soon, anyway, right?"

"Mmm-hmmm. Thank you for sending the ticket. It came in the mail today."

"I'll pick you up in Bakersfield when you fly in on Sunday."

"It'll be good to see you. Feels like forever."

"How's the rotation going?"

"It's good," I said, smiling.

Blake was silent. "Good to hear you're getting along well. You didn't sound so good last week."

"Brant's amazing. His diagnostic skills are nothing short of miraculous, and he's so helpful. Anything I need, he's always there for me, no matter how late it is. After the previous rotation," I sighed, "it's such a pleasure." My smile stretched my face so wide, I chuckled. I'd forgotten what if felt like.

"What's this guy like?"

"Pardon?"

"What's he like? Is he married?"

"What the hell kind of question is *that*? He's my resident. He's helping me. I'm getting through and it's not like having my teeth pulled every day."

Blake didn't say anything.

"You're jealous?" This was too much. Way too much.

"Damn straight, I'm jealous." Blake's voice was rough. "You never have time for me and you're spending plenty of time with other people at school."

"Studying? That's spending time?"

"And you haven't sounded so happy in months. Certainly not when I've been with you."

"Is that any surprise? You're jealous all the time, no matter what I do. Is our whole life going to be like this? I've never done anything to deserve this."

He said nothing.

"If this is the way you feel, like you can't trust me, you might as well not bother anymore." I struggled to hold back the tears. If I started crying, I'd just blubber and wouldn't be able to ask my next question. I gritted my teeth. "What I'd really like to know is, what happened to your marriage? Did your wife leave you or what?"

Silence rang through the phone lines for long moments, then Blake took a deep breath and started, his voice raising with every word. "No, I left her. She screwed around on me with my best friend. And yes, she was younger than me," he said, and hesitated, "though she was still older than you. Does that make you happy? What else do you want to know?"

I didn't know what to say. Neither of us spoke for long minutes. My anger fell away and all I felt was sorry. "No," I whispered. "I'm sorry. Nothing else."

"I'm sorry, too, Lena," Blake finally said with a groan like his guts were being wrenched out. "You're not Jana, and I have no right to put my anger with her onto you… a million times, sorry."

"Me too. There's just nothing left of me," I whispered.

"I'm afraid to lose you and I'm afraid to shut down. I just don't know what to do."

"I love you, Blake. Thanks for telling me."

"You deserved to know." Grudgingly.

"Will you be home tomorrow?" I asked.

"Not at the times you'll be home. I thought I'd try to catch up with Jordan for Christmas."

"Jordan, your son? You know where he is?"

"I found him last week. He's willing to meet with me."

"Oh Blake, that's wonderful." I hadn't heard anything so good in days.

"So Merry Christmas for tomorrow," he said gruffly.

"And to you. I'm sorry not to be there for our first Christmas."

"Me too. You go to sleep and I'll try to catch you tomorrow, okay?"

"Okay. Love you. Night night." I said as I drifted off to sleep.

"It's so good to be outside, and finally back here," said Lena, staring off across Elk Valley, as she stroked Tessa's neck.

Blake glanced at her face. Lena's tan had faded to nothing. She'd clearly spent the past several weeks indoors. He'd never seen her look like this. Happier than after her first small animal rotation, but she still hacked, even with the inhaler. "Happy to be home?"

She swallowed and didn't look back at him from her seat atop Tessa. "Yes," she said.

"Are you okay?" Blake had to ask.

She took a deep breath. "I think we just need some time to get used to each other again. Get some trust back."

"You might be right." Blake looked down into the valley beside them. "We'll have plenty of that soon, as soon as school's done."

I hope.

"What's your training schedule been for the horses?" Lena finally looked over her shoulder at him.

"We've only got another"—he counted on his fingers—"six days before the race. Today we'll go twenty miles, and tomorrow—"

Tessa whinnied frantically over a great rumbling and slithering sound, then Prince was scrambling backwards as the trail beneath his feet crumbled. When he stopped, snorting, the trail, Tessa, and Lena were gone.

Blake leapt to the ground. "*Lena!*" he yelled. "*Lena!*"

A few rocks still slid and bounced downward where the trail had been. Blake stepped toward the edge and dropped to his belly, then inched forward.

A hundred and twenty feet below, on the valley floor, Tessa was just getting to her feet and gave a great shake. As Blake watched, the mare limped through the loose rocks and boulders toward Lena, lying still as death ten yards from her.

"Lena!" he called again, but she never moved.

18

Blake shook his head, fear for Lena rising by the second as he searched the area around the slip for a safe place to get down the hillside.

No way down.

He'd have to find another way. Mounting Prince, he spun him around. From memory, there was a fire trail… yes, there. They turned onto it and scanned the valley for any movement, any help, as they raced down the trail. Nothing moved at the bottom but the gray mare, grazing wisps of grass near Lena.

Within minutes, he was at her side.

"Lena?"

She didn't answer, but she was breathing. She lay curled up on her side, covered with dust and grit, but the only blood he could see ran from a cut over a rapidly-swelling egg on her head. The helmet she'd been wearing was nowhere in sight. He made sure there was nothing in her mouth and wrapped his coat around her. "Oh my god, Lena?" he said again, but she still didn't respond.

He quickly checked Tessa. The mare was covered with dust and very lame in one forelimb but seemed otherwise intact.

Blake slipped her bridle from her head, put on her halter, and tied her to a nearby tree. With another look at Lena and a hug for the mare, he swung up on Prince and galloped to the closest house to call for a chopper.

The people were kindness itself and called the ambulance, then drove behind him back to the slide with blankets and hot water bottles.

Blake had only just dismounted and tied Prince beside Tessa when the throbbing sound of the chopper's rotors filled the air. Untying their leads, he held tightly to both skittering horses as the chopper came down.

"Blake?" shouted his friend Marcus, the chopper pilot from Bakersfield.

"Didn't waste any time, did you? Thanks for coming. She's not good at all," Blake said, biting his lip as he helped Marcus carry the stretcher towards Lena while his partner gathered more gear.

"Is this your girl?" Marcus ducked down beside her and began checking her out. Blake gave her details, as much as he knew, and Marcus introduced his partner. Together they got her strapped onto the board, and then into the stretcher. "I'm not feeling any fractures, and she appears stable, but she's got a pretty good knock on the head. Hopefully she'll be back with us soon. You coming?"

Blake glanced at the horses. The helpful neighbors had just driven away. "I need to take these guys home, then I'll drive to the hospital."

"Okay," Marcus looked dubiously at him. "See you soon. Drive safely."

They hopped into the chopper and she lifted, leaving a cloud of dust, as Blake rode the stallion and ponied the limping mare alongside them.

Blake had just finished bandaging Tessa's injured legs when

the beat-beat of a chopper came over the hill behind the house.

"Oh no, not another one," Blake said to Myrtle.

"Horses aren't the safest habit," she said, putting the sad mare's bucket down. "I hope Lena's okay, and Tessa, too." She turned to watch the chopper. "I'll finish up here. You've got to get going."

"It's Marcus, and he's landing." Blake said, recognizing the chopper. "I wonder why he's come back?" The horses snorted, but left their noses in their buckets.

"Thought you might need a ride," Marcus shouted from the chopper.

Blake gave him a thumbs up and raced to grab some clean clothes for himself and Lena. He was back in moments.

"I'll see you when you get back," Myrtle said. "Don't you worry about anything here, I've got it."

He smiled at her and gave her a quick one-armed hug, then bent over and ran under the rotors.

Marcus waved away his thanks. "If it was my woman, I'd be driving like a mad thing to get down to her. Thought it'd be safer to pick you up here than out of a crashed truck."

"Thanks, man," Blake said, shaking his head. "I owe you one."

Blake shivered at the hospital disinfectant scent as he walked in through the emergency entrance from the chopper pad. He'd spent more time than he liked within their white walls, but he was still alive.

Lena was still unconscious. He swallowed hard when the nurse showed him into Lena's curtained-off cubicle.

"We're pretty sure she has no spinal injuries," the young emergency room doctor said, "but she's had a pretty nasty knock on the head. We've sutured it, but now we just have to wait. She's young and strong. How did she do it, by the way?"

Blake told them.

"Rough. I'll be back to check on her. If there are any changes, could you please use the call button? We'll be here right away."

"Thanks, Doctor."

Blake sat in silence beside her for what felt like hours, holding her hand. Finally he had to say something.

"I'm so sorry, Lena," he whispered, gripping her fingers for grim death. "I should never have let you take the lead, not after that last landslide. I was skulking behind, letting you go ahead on a trail you barely knew.

"Please wake up. I promise I won't make you crazy anymore. I know you love me, I just need to get a handle on this jealousy. I'll love you forever. I won't be jealous of you anymore, just wake up, please?"

She stirred, the hint of a smile on her face.

"Lena?"

She opened her mouth, then shut it again. "Oh, my head… who hit me?" she finally murmured.

"A rock or a horse, not sure which," Blake said, and stood up beside her. He bent over and gently, oh so gently, kissed her lips. "The trail slipped out from under you and Tessa."

"Is Tessa okay? Prince? You?"

"We're all fine. Tess is lame, but she'll be okay."

Lena closed her eyes again. "I heard that, what you said…" Her lips shaped into a faint smile.

"And I meant it," Blake said.

"That's good… because… I'm not going… to fall down… a mountain just to hear you say that again." Lena squeezed his hand and closed her eyes. She slept.

Sleeping in the chair beside Lena's hospital bed wasn't great, but it had to be better than being in her position. By the next morning, Lena was well enough to leave.

"Excuse me, Mr. Sagan, but there's a phone call for you," a nurse said from outside the cubicle.

It was Marcus. "I'm outside. I was just coming off shift, and asked the doctor about Lena. He said she'd probably be released soon. Your chariot awaits."

"I was wondering how we would get home." Blake shook his head. "Thanks, Marcus. We'll see you in a half hour or so, as soon as they let her go."

Lena was walking around the room when he returned.

"Before you say anything"—she held up one hand—"the doctor wanted me up and walking around while they prepared the discharge papers."

"Are you sure?" he growled.

"Quite. So, Blake, no more fears, right?"

"Yes. No more stressing, right?"

Lena smiled. "Nope. And we can work on everything together?"

He nodded. "No more misunderstandings. Talking."

Blake enclosed her in his arms and held on, thankful to be given a second chance to prove his love.

Always and forever.

"I'm so sorry Tessa's hurt. That tendon should heal, but it'll take awhile," I said.

"I'm sorry too, but you're in no condition to ride in the race, anyway." Blake looked at me sadly.

"I'm fine. The doctor said I could ride. I've had no ill effects since the first day."

Blake shook his head. "I imagine he thought you were talking about a little walk around an arena, not fifty miles over rough terrain."

"I suspect I didn't make myself"—I rolled my eyes —"completely clear."

Blake brushed the hair back out of his eyes and blinked at

her. "You look good… better than good, as usual." He reached for me and I melted into his arms.

"I'm even more sorry for your injury," he said, "but it let me realize just what we mean to each other and helped us resolve some issues, anyway."

I nodded and reached up to kiss him. "I'll go make us some breakfast while you move that hay."

Ten minutes later, a crash came from the direction of the barn and both horses stood, ears pricked, staring at the barn, before they trotted over and disappeared into their stalls.

I smiled. They were probably going in for a treat. When they didn't come out again, I called down to the barn, but there was no answer.

The horses' ears were still pricked, watchful over their half-doors, all attention on the man sitting on a hay bale, swearing the sky down as he held his ribs, his face white as a sheet.

"What have you done to yourself?" I said, as I trotted to him. "Are you okay?"

"The gutter," he winced. "It blocked up a few weeks ago when it rained. Thought I'd clean it out." He wouldn't look at me.

I closed my eyes and I waited while he stalled. "What happened?" I finally asked.

"Nothing," he mumbled.

"Let me see," I said past gritted teeth, and gently pulled him to his feet. Something was clearly not right. I slowly peeled his shirt up. And gasped.

"Damned ladder tipped over," he muttered.

"Don't you know you're—" I started to berate him about old men and ladders, but I shut my mouth when I saw the line of red marks overlying several ribs, and alongside them, the hint of blue, already spreading.

"Can you breathe in for me, gently?" I asked him.

He grimaced. "Probably not." But he tried. And blanched further.

They were clearly fractured, and the race was in three days.

"It'll be better tomorrow. Fine for the race," he said, with a gasp. "They're just bruised. I've done this before. I have three more days."

I blinked.

Over my dead body, he'll be riding.

He'd *not* be riding, no matter what excuse he could find.

BLAKE'S CHEST looked much worse in the morning, but he wouldn't let me take him to the hospital.

"They'll just tape me up and tell me to rest. They usually do."

"Some X-rays would be a good idea," I growled, for the tenth time since we'd woken up.

"They're all out where I can see them. I'll take it easy," Blake argued. "We don't have time to go down there and it won't make any difference.

I quirked my lips at him.

"What?"

"Well," I said, "that was my argument last time I broke five ribs, so I guess I don't have much to say about it."

He started to laugh, stopped with a wince, then just smiled. He *carefully* pulled me closer, then let go. "It hurts too much to do even that."

I nodded, remembering how much my own ribs had ached, especially while bending over, so I kissed my fingers and touched them to his lips.

"Blake, I'm fine."

"I know you are." He looked at me sideways, his eyes narrowed, and waited for it.

"You've worked so hard getting both of these horses ready to race."

"Nothing doing, girl." Blake shook his head. "You've just come out of the hospital with head trauma, remember?"

"But I feel fine. I even called the doctor… and this time I told him what kind of riding I had in mind." I went on, as fast as I could go. "He said as long as my vision was fine and I had no dizziness or pain, I was fine to race."

He started to sigh, but froze instead, and stood still, biting his lip, then turned concerned eyes on me. "You've never even been *on* Prince."

"I could ride him. He knows me."

"He's a stallion. Anything could happen."

"I've handled plenty of stallions."

"In a race, with a hundred other horses, on narrow trails?"

"I promise, I'll keep him away from everyone."

"It'll only end in tears."

"It'll be fine. And if I don't feel fine, or if I get worried, I'll pull him."

He stood leaning against the kitchen doorjamb in silence for long minutes. "Okay," he finally murmured. "I don't want to risk you again, but if you're dead set on doing it and truly feel fine, it may be possible to switch Prince's rider with the race committee."

Blake was as good as his word. He called and left a message for Leslie, the ride manager, and she rode up to talk with us soon afterwards.

"Sure, we can switch Prince's rider, and I already have your details, Lena." She smiled at me. "I'll pull Miś Witeża. I heard about what happened, and she's clearly lame now," Leslie said, with a glance over her shoulder at the mare, "so you don't even need a vet certificate."

That was rather decent of her. "Thank you for that, Leslie."

"I don't know what's going on but everyone's getting broken. Have you heard about Dr. Morton?"

"No, what's up?" He frowned.

"She fell off her horse yesterday."

"Is she okay?" Blake cringed at his sharp intake of breath.

"She broke her leg, but otherwise, she's okay. She won't be vetting the ride, though. We're hustling to find another vet in time, but we'll manage. Luckily, we still have Seth, our head vet, but he can't do it alone." She backed her horse away from the porch. "I'm off. You take care of yourself, eh? See you at the race."

I LOOKED up at the sky, clear blue without a hint of cloud, as I finished checking Prince's shoes for any loose nails one final time. "Lovely day for the race. I'm sorry you can't ride Prince today," I said as I walked over to Blake, "but I'll do my best to take care of him for you."

"Well"—Blake grimaced as he picked up a bucket, swallowed hard, and straightened up—"at least I can crew for you two."

I shook my head. "Marcus said for you to leave the buckets. He'll be right back." I kissed him on the lips. Gently. "Are you sure you want to do this? We could get you a job pushing paper at one of the registration desks. I don't know how you're going to stand the drives between vet checks."

"Easy." He twisted his lips. "I'll drive. The ribs are better with a steering wheel in my hands."

He had a point. From experience, I knew it was a good one.

"Blake," called a girl on a bay Morgan, "have you heard about the pre-rides?"

"We did it last night, Maria," he said. "Didn't you?"

"Yes, but for some reason the head vet says the new vet they just pulled in wants to see the horses himself, so they're doing another pre-ride vet check."

"Can they do that?"

"I don't know"—the girl shrugged—"but they're doing it."

I looked at Blake. "Well, do we front up for it?"

"If Maria says that's what they're doing, I guess so. Can you bring Prince along?" he said, and stiffly made his way toward the vet check area.

Prince was good at his job, and he knew it was race day. All ready to start the race, he danced on the end of his lead until Blake growled at him, then he settled.

The new vet stood talking to one of the competitors. Something about his stance niggled at my brain, sending a shiver up my spine, but I shook my head and looked down to negotiate some rocks in our path. We were nearly to the enclosure when the vet turned around and I saw his face—and froze.

"Lena, are you okay?" Blake's voice seemed to come from far away. "Lena, what's the matter? You're white as a sheet."

My world was going gray and I gulped air like a guppy. "Blake," I whispered, as his arm came around me, "it's him."

19

"Who?" Blake's brows narrowed, and he stared at the crowd assembled at the gate to the vet check.

"The new vet—he's the one from school"—I breathed against his shirt—"my nemesis—"

Blake spun toward the vet with a sharp intake of breath. He locked his jaw and slowly breathed out. "So, that's the jerk."

I nodded. "Gareth Barnett-Payne. I wouldn't put anything past him. He's the devil incarnate," I said, as I frayed the end of Prince's leadrope with both hands. "Can you keep your eyes peeled for me, please?" I tasted bile in my throat and swallowed hard to keep it down.

"Hold on, Lena. He can't do anything with all these people here."

I raised a brow at him and tried to stop shaking as I led Prince forward.

By the stare he sent my way, Gareth expected me, no question about that. There wasn't a hint of surprise in his steely eyes. I could have sworn I heard Blake growl from behind me.

Just before I reached the in-gate, Blake called out to me. "Lena, the head vet needs a ride to the first stop right now. You going to be okay?" He turned a baleful look toward Gareth.

I nodded, though I knew it was impossible to be okay with Gareth Barnett-Payne in the same county.

Blake winced over his shoulder at me but followed the official who was practically tugging at his sleeve. "See you there," he shouted, and his brow furrowed as he waved.

"Lena Scott?" Gareth said, checking his secretary's clipboard, then handing it back to her. "What have we here?" He looked Prince over, then asked me to trot him out.

His eyes burned a hole in my back as I jogged away, Prince bouncing along beside me, stopped, turned, and trotted back toward him, my eyes on a spot somewhere beyond him. Looking at Gareth wasn't helping my sanity.

"You're nearly a vet, Lena. How could you do this to a horse?"

I blinked. "Pardon?"

"He's totally out of condition."

I shook my head. "He's a stallion. I thought the same the first time I saw him, too, but it's all muscle."

He raised a brow at me and shook his head. "He's too fat. He'll get into trouble in the race. You should know that." Flatly.

"There's not an ounce of superfluous fat on this horse. It's all stallion muscle. Truly." I closed my eyes for a second. "Please? Let us start, and you'll see. He already passed the pre-ride last night. Dr. Latimer didn't have a problem with him."

"Well, I do."

"Please?" I was pleading now, and something changed in his eyes—he almost smiled. *Bastard.* Pleading women, his favorite. I gritted my teeth.

Gareth stood in silence for a moment. Finally, with a glint

in his eye, he agreed to let Prince start. "I'll be waiting at the second vet check to pull you if he's not in perfect health." His jaw tight, he took a step toward me, evil in his eyes, but Prince snaked his head around toward him, teeth bared. Gareth stopped in his tracks and glared at the pair of us.

"He'll be okay," I murmured. Damned if I was going to thank him.

"Passed," he said, through clenched teeth, to his secretary. "Next?" he called out, and we bolted.

I looked for Blake, but all I saw were his tail lights heading off toward the first vet check.

My vision cleared again as I bridled Prince and told Marcus what was up. The chopper pilot offered the horse another drink of electrolyte water and saddled him. I made sure Prince's hoof boot was lashed firmly to his saddle, retrieved my rider card and ID from the trailer, and stowed them in my pack. I smiled as I returned to the fidgety stallion, looking at our competitor number. Thirteen, my lucky number, was marked in a fluoro-orange livestock paint stick on his left hip. It suited him—the horse might just get a saddle pad of the same color for his birthday. With that color marking his flank, at least they could find us if he was unlucky enough to slide down the side of a mountain.

Then the five-minute warning was called, and everything was a flurry. Marcus gave me a leg up and sent me on my way. "I'll see you at the vet check," he yelled after me.

Per Blake's instructions, I held Prince, the only stallion in the race, off to one side of the starting line. No use creating a scene or getting anyone hurt. He quivered as he waited for the gun to go, and then we were off.

Thankfully, I knew the course fairly well, after riding the start area for several days. Knowing there was plenty of room for several horses abreast in the first few miles helped. I let Prince settle into his long trot that ate up the miles. When he was out moving, he tended to think of his work, and not of the girls around him. Several horses took off at a canter and passed us, but Prince, other than a brief flick of his little ears, ignored them. I suspect he knew he'd pass them soon.

Five miles out, we did. He trotted along, looking neither right nor left, and already, we were passing horses which had started out too fast. By the time we reached a narrower trail, there were only a handful of horses in front of us.

My heart sang. To be blessed with riding such a horse… he seemed to be in his element in competition. All I needed to do was think "forward", and he flew.

Like all good endurance horses, especially on the longer rides such as the Tevis, Prince drank when there was water and nibbled at any available grass he could reach while trotting past. The horses that stayed well-hydrated and kept their guts going stayed well—and performed well.

We must have been nearly to the ten-mile mark when a trough showed beside the trail ahead. Prince headed for it and plunged his whole muzzle beneath the surface, then lifted his head and shook it. When he returned his lips to the surface and began to drink, I counted the swallows going down his esophagus. Good drinker he was, but I wouldn't founder him by letting him have too much water.

One, two, three, four, five, six—one liter, two, three, four, five, six—two liter…

Prince flung up his head and spun around, every muscle tense as he tested the air. A little brown Arabian sporting four white socks with an older woman aboard planted her feet and whinnied shrilly to Prince. The filly backed up a few steps, but her rider kicked her on and pushed her forward.

"Is she on heat?" I called to the woman and took a firmer grip on Prince's reins.

"Yes, she is," she said.

"This is a stallion. Could you please take her around to the other side, or wait? We'll be done in a moment."

The woman glared at me and jerked the filly hard to the left, and around toward the other side of the trough, but the filly began backing again, then stopped, spread her hind legs, and urinated in little squirts.

Prince's throaty stallion whicker vibrated through his whole body, and out to my legs, but he remained obedient to the reins.

The woman prodded her forward again, this time toward the trough and us, snarling at her horse and, I suspect, at me. The filly stepped forward, then leapt into the trough with both forefeet to get to Prince, whinnying at the top of her lungs as the woman started to shriek.

I backed Prince away, which didn't impress him. He stuffed his head down to buck, but I managed to drive him on, pushing him hard to the right, away from the floundering filly. When we reached the edge of the clearing, I glanced back at the ruckus to make sure they were okay.

The rider had dismounted and tugged the filly out of the plastic trough. Thankfully, I saw no flashes of red on her white stockings.

"Stallions and people who ride them shouldn't be in races," she ranted, at full noise.

Funny, she hadn't added in-heat mares to her list.

"Sorry," I called, just for good measure, and we bolted.

"Good boy, Prince," I said, shakily, and patted his neck. That could've ended badly. If Prince were any less well-behaved... it mightn't have been pretty at all.

Soon we were into the first vet check, and Blake was beside me in an instant, gripping my leg. I slid from Prince's saddle and handed him to Marcus to walk cool. Blake wasn't impressed when I gave him the lowdown on Gareth and on the lady at the trough.

"That man needs to be reported." He didn't even mention the trough incident. Clearly, it was a lesser concern.

"He's evil, Blake. Let's see if we can get through this without a direct confrontation," I begged.

"Thankfully, he's not at this check. He'll be at the next one, though. We'll stick close, never you worry, darlin'."

Prince passed through the check with flying colors when his hold time was up and we were away again.

As I had been from the start of the race, I hopped off and ran the downhills to save Prince's legs. It was easy for me and would probably make a big difference to him over time. It *was* a beautiful day, and I wasn't about to let that creep Gareth destroy it for me, no matter how hard he tried.

With the morning's progress, the temperature rose. It was going to be a scorcher. I kept hydrated from my water bottles and Prince drank from every small spring we passed.

AT THE SECOND VET CHECK, Blake and Marcus flanked me as Gareth checked Prince's vitals. The vet scowled and gritted his teeth, but he couldn't find fault with the horse beneath his stethoscope, even if he didn't like the rider. He looked at Prince doubtfully, but by his recovery, he had no real excuse to pull him.

With a kiss of Blake's lips, I mounted up again and was walking toward the exit gate when I glanced in Gareth's direction just in time to see the filthy look Gareth flung in Blake's direction. I expected that. It wasn't a surprise.

What *did* bother me, though, was the grin of malicious delight that followed, as he continued to look at Blake.

Not a good sign.

I nearly lost my seat when Prince was bumped from behind. He leapt forward and spun toward whatever had just hit him. A flash of brown and white and the heavy thud of two hind hooves meeting flesh, and my world exploded in a flash of pain.

Through a blur of tears, I pulled Prince back and away from the direction of whatever horse had just blasted us and glanced up to see the brown Arab filly. Again. I swore a blue streak at shriek level and reached down to grip my ankle. Her silly owner, red-faced, had just caught up the horse's leadrope. She tugged for all she was worth while the filly pulled to get away and back to Prince.

"Get that filly out of here, you idiot," Blake yelled at her as he raced toward me, his face stormy. "Holy crap, Lena, are you okay?" He made it to my side in seconds and pulled me out of the saddle, ribs or no ribs.

I didn't trust my voice to do anything but swear some more, so I only nodded.

"Is that the cow with the filly from the trough?" he demanded.

"Yes," I spat, with a glare in her direction.

"Marcus, can you pick her up and take her back to the truck? I'll take the horse and go get some ice," Blake said, and added his own string of curses.

"I'll be okay," I said, as I tried to put weight on the leg, and quickly jerked it off the ground.

Blake frowned at me. "You're done. I heard that kick. You'll be a toast by the next check. I'll be right back. You're done," he repeated, and hurried on ahead.

Marcus picked me up like a small sack of—breakable—potatoes and made his way back to the truck.

"Marcus, can you get me the bandages in the tack box?" I said softly in to his ear, wincing as my bad ankle bumped into the other one. "And a bigger boot? There's a pair in the camper."

He turned his head to me. "What do you have in mind?"

"I'm going on."

"Can I watch?" he whispered dryly. "Blake won't take it sitting down."

"I'll be fine. I'll wrap it up snugly and it'll be okay. I'm sure it's not broken."

"And how, miss vet, do you know that?"

"When I move it around, there's no *crepitus*."

"In English."

"It doesn't crunch and gronch."

He shuddered.

"Will you help me? I probably could use something rigid, like a bit of flat wood? Two pieces?"

"He's not going to let you."

"If it's bandaged before he gets back, he will."

"Your funeral, girl."

Marcus stalked off, shaking his head, but he found what I needed. I had the already grossly swollen and blue-green tinged ankle wrapped up with elastic sticky bandage, sticks cunningly padded and wrapped in place, long before Blake returned with the ice.

I stood and put some weight on the contraption.

"If you get any whiter, you'll pass out," Marcus observed. "Here he comes."

"What are you doing on that leg? Sit down and put it up," Blake growled as he reached us.

"It's okay. Just bruised. I've wrapped it up and I'm ready to go on. I don't have much time." I glanced at my watch. "I was supposed to leave two minutes ago." I bent to pull my tights down over the bandage and strap on the half-chaps, grateful I was riding in them, rather than breeches.

"You can't be serious," Blake said with a frown.

"I've had worse. I can live with it." I bit my lips together. And the anti-inflammatories I'd just tossed back should kick in soon, too.

"I heard that impact. Prince is okay, thankfully, but—"

"I'm okay to go, really. Look, I'll even tape that ice onto it," I said, as I reached for it.

Blake stood glaring. "You can't possibly ride like that."

"I can. Please? We're late already."

He shook his head and looked at me doubtfully. "If you really think it's okay…"

"I do. Can you give me a lift please? This leg's a bit heavy." A grin cracked through my tight lips.

"I really don't feel good—"

"I'll be fine. Kiss me so we can get out of here," I said. His lips, tight, met mine, and I spun the horse around and we headed off at a trot, watching all around for wayward fillies.

It wasn't long before I had to drop my stirrups and flip them over Prince's withers. Like just around the corner from the vet check, out of Blake's sight. There'd be no running the downhills for me for the rest of this race. Trotting wasn't a good option, either. For all my assurances, I had no idea if there was a fracture. I just knew I had to finish this race… for my Nonna. She didn't get to finish her big race… and would never have the chance again.

Ever.

20

The day just got hotter and hotter.

"I'm worried about Lena," Blake said, to Marcus, as he wiped the sweat from his brow. "Not only can she barely walk, and that's bad news if something more happens out on the trail, but that guy's cruisin' for a bruisin', messing with her like that."

Marcus gave him a wry grin. "And you're not the one who's going to give it to him. Lena'll have to do that herself."

Blake glared at his friend. "She's in no way big enough, and she's hurt."

"She has another way to do it. One we can't touch."

Blake took the deepest breath he could without screaming in pain and turned back toward the gap in the trees through which the horses would come. "They're sitting on third place. I wonder if she knows?"

"I doubt it. She's just focused on taking care of your horse." Marcus smiled. "She's a good girl, that."

"Don't I know it," Blake murmured and frowned at the leadrope he held in his hands.

"What's the matter?"

"You know about Jana, right?"

Marcus nodded.

"I can't let it go."

"Let what go?"

"Believing it's not going to happen again. And I'm driving Lena crazy with it."

"Is she messing around on you?"

"No," he said, and closed his eyes. When he opened them, Marcus was frowning.

"Then what's the problem?" Marcus said, his brows nearly touching.

"I can't seem to get over it and trust her. But soon it'll be okay. She'll be down here, and I won't have anything to worry about."

The chopper pilot was silent. When Blake turned to face him, Marcus was slowly shaking his head at him, incredulity in his eyes.

"What?" Blake demanded.

"Location makes no difference."

"Of course, it does," Blake said, glaring.

"Did it make a difference last time?"

Blake barely heard the whispered question from his friend, but he pretended he hadn't. It would be fine.

It had to be.

"Are we all ready for Lena to come in?" he asked Marcus. "I feel useless, not even able to carry buckets."

"That's what I'm here for, remember?"

He nodded. "Thanks for listening. I'll get through it, and it'll all be a—"

"Number thirteen!" the gatekeeper shouted.

They spun toward the gate to see Lena trot in.

"How's the leg?" Blake asked, as he reached out to pull her from the saddle and winced even before his hands got to her waist. He gritted his teeth and stepped closer.

"Blake, I can get down myself, you're going to hurt your—"

"Let me help," Marcus said, stepping closer.

"It's not gonna kill me." Blake ignored Marcus. "But watching you hit the ground and scream might," he growled and wrapped his arms around my waist.

"Blake, let Marc—" Lena snapped, as Blake, not as gently as he might have, tugged.

She bit back the scream as her ankle dragged over Prince's saddle and Blake swore as Lena clawed the heck out of his arm with her fingernails, and probably wrecked what was left of his ribs, but she was finally down on *terra firma*.

They both glanced back at Marcus.

The chopper pilot stood, one brow raised and mustache quirked to one side. He raised his hands. "I'm not sayin' anything. You clearly have it all under control." He chuckled and turned to walk Prince away for a drink.

Lena and Blake looked at each other.

"Sorry," they both said at the same time, and both winced their way back to the trailer.

"It's tough, trotting this far without stirrups, I let him lope as much as he felt like," Lena said, swallowing hard. "This horse is magic, though."

Prince pushed his nose against Marcus, who gave him a scratch while he drank. The stallion munched a few mouthfuls of hay while Lena had a drink of water and a snack bar.

"You can't go on like this," Blake said past gritted teeth.

She ignored him. "There's plenty of water out there," Lena said as Blake checked Prince's membranes and pulled the skin over the point of his shoulder. "He's drinking well at every chance and he's still nibbling any grass or bushes within reach. He's the best endurance horse I've ever ridden."

Blake looked at her. "He looks fantastic, but you don't."

"It's probably all the dirt." She gave him a cheeky grin.

Blake sighed. She wasn't going to give an inch. "Prince's probably glad not to have to lug me around. I'm sure I've got fifty pounds on you," he said, "stirrups or no stirrups." He ducked down beside her. "Lena, I'm serious. If that leg's broken—"

"It's not broken. I can stand on it."

"If it were a spiral fracture, you might still be able to."

"But I'm okay."

"Why are you so dead set on staying in the race? There'll be other races, but if you wreck that ankle now, you might not *get* to do them later."

She looked at him, her jaw set in frustration and tears in her eyes.

Whoa. What have we here?

"Remember," she whispered, "when I told you about my grandma? The one who was training, but didn't get to do that Tevis because she was so sick from cancer?"

Blake gripped her hand tightly and nodded.

"Well, this is for her. After I was kicked, and I thought I'd quit, I realized I couldn't. This is for Nonna."

"She wouldn't want you to go through this much pain."

"This is for *her*. Unless you pull the horse, I'm going through with it," she said, through clenched jaws.

"Well then," Blake said, "guess you're goin' on."

Marcus came over, probably seeing we'd stopped growling at each other.

"Should we tell her, or should we make her wait?" Marcus grinned at Blake.

He took a deep breath and glared at Marcus.

Lena brushed at her leaky eyes and frowned. "Tell me what?" She looked from one to the other.

"You're holding third place," Blake muttered, "but it's not worth risking yourself for."

Her eyes bugged. "*Really?*" She struggled to her feet and

threw her arms around Prince's neck. "I knew you were magic," she mumbled into his long mane.

"Now just because you're placing, don't go gettin' cocky, just *try* to take care of yourself and your horse and… I hope everything'll be fine." Blake tried to smile, but he was past it. All he could do was roll his eyes and clamp his jaws together.

Letting go of the horse, Lena held Blake by the shoulders and kissed him. "Good thing I can hug the horse. You'd be screaming if I tried to hug you," she said, as she slipped the girth and started to slide Prince's saddle off. "Really, Blake, I'll be okay," she murmured at him as he took her hands off the saddle and removed it himself.

Blake fed her while Marcus walked Prince, and then they were back in the vet box with Dr. Latimer. Marcus ran beside Prince for the trot-out, and soon Prince and Lena were trotting out of the rest stop.

She was worth getting a few things sorted in his head… if they both lived through this race.

He'd do it.

He had no other choice.

"Woo hoo!" Lena shrieked, as she passed the finish line! "We did it, Prince!"

"You sure did, honey," said the woman taking her number and her rider card. "Well done. You just go on over there and the P & R team will write down your numbers."

"Thank you," she called back.

"Congratulations, Lena," Blake said, held his breath, gritted his teeth, and hugged her, then let his breath out slowly. Despite her excitement, Lena's face was white as a sheet.

"Thank you so much for letting me ride him. He's a gem,"

she said as Marcus helped her off again. He buckled his halter around Prince's neck and slipped his bridle off, while Lena reached for the carrot Marcus held out to her.

"Congratulations, girl! You took good care of that horse. He looks like a million bucks," Marcus said.

Prince bit the carrot and munched contentedly, then took the rest of it and played with it in his water bucket.

"We passed someone," Lena said excitedly, as she hopped a few steps to hand Prince's bridle to Blake.

"You sure did. You're second."

Lena gazed between him and the horse with stars in her eyes. "I just can't believe it. What a horse. I'm sure you'll get tired of me saying that for the next few days." She grinned.

"Never. He *is* that good. Now let's go get him ready for the post-ride check."

With another hug around the stallion's neck, Lena led him away to nibble grass and cool down. Blake handed her a stethoscope and she checked him.

"He's coming right down and his color's great. Not a lick of dehydration."

"Proud of you, girl," Blake said as he took her hand and walked along with her, "but you need to get off that leg. The horse looks great, but you"—he glanced down to see her grimace—"look like crap." He kept Lena turned toward him, so she never saw Barnett-Payne walking toward them. Over her shoulder, Blake challenged the creep with his best stare. The vet must have decided he didn't really want to torture her… not just yet.

Soon, their time was up, and they headed for the vet check.

"Thank you, again, Blake, for everything," Lena said, her eyes aglow. He squeezed her hand and let her and the stallion go, her limping, but him looking fantastic, off into the taped-off post-ride control vet check.

An official asked Lena her name and glanced at her watch, then noted something on her clipboard. She indicated where Lena and Prince were to wait then moved on to the next horse.

Blake turned his attention to the first-place horse, currently being examined by the vets. Two members of the P & R team were walking away from the horse toward the vets, frowning. Even from here, Blake could see the gray was lame at a walk in one foreleg. There were hard, gaunt lines over his flanks and rump and his coat was staring. Even when he stood still, he appeared a little unsteady on his feet. When he trotted out, his head bobbed over his left fore. Blake bit his lip and shook his head.

"What's going on?" Marcus murmured.

"That rider's not in a good position. AERC's motto is 'To Finish is to Win'. The corollary of that is that unless a horse is deemed 'ready to go on', it isn't a finisher, much less a winner."

"Oh. How disappointing for him. I suspect he went too fast to try to win."

"I wasn't out on the trail, so I can't comment, but it's a possibility."

They watched as the vets both took turns listening to his heart and lungs, then they stepped away to confer. The P & R team joined them.

"Not fit to continue," Dr. Latimer called out to the official, whose brows narrowed as she wrote on her clipboard. "Disqualified."

The P & R team approached Lena and Prince and started taking his vitals. They'd just turned to their secretary when Gareth interrupted them and seemed to take over. They watched the vet glare at the team and they slowly backed off, while he turned back to Prince and started examining the horse.

"What about the P & R team?" Marcus turned to Blake with a frown.

"I don't know. I don't like the look of this." Blake swore beneath his breath.

Lena said something to Gareth and her face blanched even whiter than it already was, as white as Blake's knuckles on the fence rail.

"The bastard. I'm going to help her."

"No, you aren't," Marcus growled low. "She can handle it."

"No, she can't," Blake muttered. "You should have seen her before. She can't handle him, and she can barely walk on that blasted leg. You've never even been to an endurance race."

"I'm here to help you both," Marcus said, past clenched teeth.

"I'm going in to—"

Marcus grabbed his arm, just as he was about to climb over the fence. "I may not have been to an endurance race, but I know how competitions work. Leave it. You'll just get her disqualified," he hissed. "Back off and let her handle it."

MY HEART SANK for the rider at the announcement disqualifying the previously-winning pair, but tingles started up in my spine, just the same.

The P & R team came over to us and one counted Prince's respiratory rate while another placed her stethoscope against Prince's chest to listen to his heart. They'd counted, and one had opened his mouth to give the secretary his results, when Gareth walked up with a smarmy look on his face. I glanced up to see Doc Latimer walking away toward the other end of the trot-up area, and my guts knotted up.

"I'll take over here, thanks," he said, and took my rider card from the secretary, who frowned.

She stood there, as did the P & R pair, but he gave them a cold smile and turned his back.

"He's looking pretty tired," Gareth said casually, when they were all out of earshot. "Doesn't look fit to go on."

Prince snorted at him and backed up, ears laid back. The horse never forgot an attitude.

"The P & R team didn't get a chance to record Prince's parameters," I said.

"That's okay. I'll do it. I have time."

The world began to spin around me, but I gritted my teeth and forced myself to stay focused.

This isn't about me.

I took a deep breath and held it, and my ground.

He's like this with all women.

"This horse is fine." My voice sounded loud to my ears and the crowd hushed. "I had to hold him in for the past mile because he knew he was coming into the finish." I shifted my weight off of my bad ankle, hoping no one would see it.

"I don't know," Gareth, shaking his head.

With some hesitation, he stepped up to the horse's shoulder and placed his stethoscope against the Prince's girth.

I ran my fingers up to the stallion's jugular and counted while he listened to his stethoscope.

Under forty-eight beats per minute.

No way was he going to pull this horse.

"His heart rate is still pretty high. He's not fit to go on and I'm going to pull him," Gareth said, with that awful look I knew so well. His "control look".

"Look, Gareth, we went to the same veterinary school." I spoke softly, but he flinched at the edge of steel I managed to put into it. "Since when does a heart rate of fifty-six equate to 'over sixty-four'?"

He glared at me. "I don't see a stethoscope on you."

"Who needs a stethoscope? Any untrained person can count a pulse," I said, then added, more softly. "Your personal life has nothing to do with this horse's fitness. Please let it go."

He spun and stomped away toward his truck.

I turned to Doc Latimer, who looked from Gareth to me, and back again, with a frown marring his face. I motioned to him to come to me, while I chewed at my lip.

"Now look, Lena, I don't know what you said to him, but the control judges are the last word on this ride, you know that. I'm sorry, but the fact you're nearly through vet school doesn't hold any water here."

21

I took a deep breath before answering the head vet. "Doc Latimer, I understand your position, but would you please check Prince's heart rate and tell me what it is?"

"Hasn't Gareth already done that, and the P & R team?"

I gritted my teeth. "He disregarded the P & R team and made them go away after they'd assessed Prince. Then he took my card away from them." I took a deep breath to steady myself. "I'm counting fifty-six. Gareth is counting it as 'over' and wants to disqualify me, though he didn't say what heart rate he'd actually counted." I gulped.

His frown deepened. "Now why would he do a thing like that? That's crazy talk, Lena."

I shuddered. I'd have to say it. "We, unfortunately, have a history… and not a salubrious one, at that."

The vet's visage softened, and he let out a breath.

And counted.

"Fifty-four." His eyes narrowed at me. "You're telling me the truth?"

I nodded. "Never been more truthful," I murmured.

Doc Latimer set his jaw and turned toward Barnett-Payne.

We all watched Gareth as he returned from his vehicle, his face thunderous.

Doc Latimer turned toward him and headed his way, then stopped and returned to Prince. He listened to his heart and lungs and noted the parameters to his secretary. "Can you trot him?"

I bit my lip. "Does the rider have to be 'able to go on' for us to complete the race?"

His mustache quirked. "Nope." He turned toward the P & R team which had just left me. "Jeff? Can I see you for a moment please?"

One young man from the P & R team came at a run.

"Jeff, can you please trot him out for us? Lena's had a bit of an injury."

"No problem, Doc," he said, and smiled at me as he took Prince's lead.

"Jeff's shown Arab stallions. Prince won't give him any trouble," he said, in response to my worried look. "You go get off that leg," he whispered.

I took a few steps away, but I wasn't going far. Jeff trotted him, turned him on his hind end, then tried to trot him straight back, but he was so full of himself that he bucked and bounced all the way back to the vet, or vets, now. Jeff came toward me with the stallion as I watched Gareth, who stood beside Doc Latimer not saying much, his jaw clenched.

As the vets began to converse again, Gareth's face grew redder and redder, then he turned away completely.

"SOUND," Doc Latimer barked, with a huge smile. "Congratulations to our new first-place winners, Prince Witeż and Lena Scott!"

From force of habit, I couldn't help watching Gareth from the corners of my eyes. He flinched as the crowd erupted and his whole body went rigid.

I dragged my attention away from him and limped Prince

back toward the truck, amidst congratulations from all around. Blake made his way to my side, took Prince's lead, and kissed me, while Prince nudged at his back.

"Well done, Lena! I'm so proud of you. Not only for the ride, but especially for standing up for yourself to him." He flicked a glance in Gareth's direction. "I thought I needed to save you, but you and Marcus proved me wrong." He pulled me against him to take some pressure off my bad leg, while somehow managing his ribs. "You can thank Marcus for keeping me on the other side of the fence."

I smiled at the beaming Marcus and returned my attention to Blake. "It's true," I said. "I couldn't have done it before. I guess I'm stronger than I was. Certainly, stronger than I thought."

"Now let's go pretty up this horse," Blake said, and kissed me again.

AN HOUR LATER, a crowd had assembled for the Best Condition trot-out and Prince and Marcus led the parade around the fenced-off area.

"That horse looks the same as he did before the race this morning," I heard one woman say to another as I stood behind the tape with Blake. "And that vet tried to pull him. No accounting for taste."

I smiled and looked up at Blake. The woman was right. Prince looked so ready to go on. "Pity about the rider," I mumbled into Blake's shirt, and he chuckled and held me snugly against his side.

My heart pounded as they worked their way through the lineup from tenth place toward us, both vets examining, and then watching the horse trot away and back. Finally, it was

Prince's turn. Prince nuzzled Doc Latimer but kept one wary eye upon Gareth whenever he was near.

"I hope Marcus can keep him from biting or kicking Gareth. He tried, you know."

Blake's brows narrowed. "That'd be a disaster."

The vets examined him thoroughly, listened to his heart and lungs twice, and then went away to confer. I squeezed Blake's hand and nodded at the three P & R team members whom Gareth had sent away from Prince and me. As one, they stalked over to the vets and Doc Latimer turned to talk with them, while Gareth's face turned stony. The trio soon retreated, and the vets resumed their discussion.

A ripple of sound spread through the assembled spectators as the two vets, voices raised, conferred back and forth. They eventually returned, both grim-faced, and handed their clipboards to the ride manager.

"Well, that's us," Blake said, one arm over Prince's back as he led him back to the trailer. "We couldn't have made him look any better than he already does."

"Thank you both for crewing today. It's a big job, lugging everything around from one stop to the next. I appreciate it from the bottom of my heart," I said after we'd put Prince into his pen. I hopped over to pick up a rubber grooming mitt to give the stallion an extra scratch.

"No problem," the guys both said, smiling at me, as Marcus took the mitt and Blake placed me in one chair and put my leg up onto another one. I had to be the luckiest girl in the world. The horse, the man… life was good.

"Congratulations again, Lena," Blake said, as they curled up together on his big bed in the top of the camper for a rest while they waited for the awards ceremony. "Despite neglecting yourself"—he frowned at her—"you took good care of the horse."

"Mmmm..." she murmured, nearly asleep. "Thank you again, but you know what?"

"What?" he dropped a kiss on the top of her head, probably one of the only places that didn't hurt.

"Remember when I thought you were a softie for having a camper?"

"Mmmm?"

"Well," she mumbled, "it's okay. Camping like this would be fine with m..."

Blake smiled. Tucking her arm beneath the covers, he pulled her against him and let sleep claim him, too.

Despite the anti-inflammatories and the nap, my ankle was worse by the time the Best Condition award was to be announced.

"I wish I could carry you, Lena," Blake said, frowning.

"Well, you can't," I said. "And Marcus has been dragging buckets for me all day. I can walk a few hundred feet." I smiled at them both.

Half an hour into the ceremony, I was called up for First Prize.

"I feel like a little kid," I said with a grin, showing Blake and Marcus the trophy.

"You earned it, sweetie," Blake said, with a smile.

The air hummed with excitement as the Best Condition prize was announced.

"And for our last prize of the day, a prize I value more than even First Place," said Doc Latimer, "because this is the prize for the person who has trained their horse carefully and taken the best care of their horse during the ride. Today I'm pleased to present this to a team who's been plagued with injuries but has done what it took to make it happen."

Blake looked over at me and my face heated.

"This horse was to be ridden by its owner, who broke his ribs three days ago, so his partner, who'd never even been on him, took the ride."

Now I was grinning fit to split. Blake squeezed my hand so hard I thought he'd break it.

"And today, after she was kicked by an on-heat mare who'd taken aim at the stallion, she bandaged her leg up and rode the rest of the race without stirrups. And still took fantastic care of this horse. If this team doesn't deserve this award today, I don't know who does."

The crowd was on its feet, facing us and applauding.

"Best Condition goes to," Doc Latimer shouted over the crowd, "our first-place winners, Lena Scott and Prince Witeż!"

Blake, wincing, gave me a big hug, then released me so I could go up front to pick up my, or rather, *our* trophy, and a hug from Doc Latimer.

Gareth was nowhere to be seen.

"Let's load up and get you to the hospital," Blake said, and drew me to my feet after the last of the riders and crews had offered their congratulations and headed for their own trucks.

"I'm okay. We need to get Prince home and bandaged, then we can go.

Blake stared at me in stony silence. "Hospital."

"Horse."

"Lena, how *about*"—Blake glared at me—"I take you to the hospital, leave you there to get X-rayed, then *I'll* take him home, get him bandaged, then come back to get you."

I sighed. I was too tired to argue anymore. "Okay," I said,

and we packed up, or rather, the men packed up after they managed to get me to sit down and put my leg up.

SOMEHOW THERE WAS no one else waiting to see the doctor at the emergency room, so Blake stayed outside to keep an eye on Prince while I saw the doctor and had my ankle X-rayed. The doctor spoke soothingly about sprains, keeping my leg elevated, and staying off it for several days.

"And please get it re-checked in a few weeks to make sure there aren't any spiral or other undisplaced fractures."

"I can do that, thank you, Doctor Parker," I said.

"I'm still astonished at how swollen it is, for not being fractured," he murmured, looking sideways at me as he held open the front door.

I smiled at him and waved as I kept walking.

"He was surprised at the amount of swelling," I said to Blake, as he helped me into the truck.

"I'm so glad it's not broken. I'd feel even worse for letting you go on with it." Blake sighed. "And I'd imagine you didn't tell him just why there was so much swelling."

"Well," I winced, "no, but it'd have been worse if I hadn't bandaged it."

Blake pursed his lips and shook his head. "I'm glad you're okay, anyway, you little minx."

Blake padded the dashboard with some towels. "Here, you settle back and get comfortable. I'm sure you could use some shut-eye, after the day you've had."

I must have dozed, and when I looked up, Blake glanced across at me and took my hand in his. I smiled lazily at him across the cab. "If I feel this stiff, I can't imagine what Prince feels like, but it's worth it. That was a fantastic—"

Blake hit the brakes as he glanced in the rear-view mirror

and I struggled toward an upright position as he eased the camper and trailer off the side of the road on a sharp corner in the four-lane highway. "Pray no one hits us. I'll get some flares," he said.

"What is it?" I sat up and my mouth dropped open at the sight of the piled-up carnage spread out in the road ahead.

"Accident." Blake's jaw was set and his face pale. "I'm not going to park any closer. Let's go. If you can, grab some blankets from the camper, and don't get hit," he barked.

I slid down from the truck just as he flicked the seat back forward and scrabbled behind it, then limped to the camper, climbed in, and dragged out the bedding.

Blake had lit a flare and set it on the road. He handed the rest to another motorist then grabbed most of my bundle and my hand, and I hopped beside him at a run for the disaster.

We split up, calling out to the people in the cars, but few answered. Those who did were already screaming. I nearly screamed myself at the pools of blood and body parts scattered on the pavement. We gave wide berth to several cars, already fiery infernos—nothing we could do to help there. The wreckage, the screams, the reek of burning rubber, and the pervasive metallic scent of blood. We struggled to pull people from their cars without damaging them further and get them away from the vehicles, vehicles in danger of catching fire along with the others, and hand them over to others who'd stopped to help.

"Has anyone gone to find a phone?" Blake shouted over the fracas. "Has an ambulance been called?"

"I've radioed for help on my CB," one man shouted, as he passed, a crying, bloody child in his arms.

The night seemed to go on forever, out on this lonely stretch of twisting road.

I COULDN'T FIND any more people to pull from the non-burning cars. My throat ached, my ankle throbbed, and my eyes burned. The smell of burning plastic and the coppery scent of blood was almost unbearable. I turned to find Blake, but he wasn't there. I limped from one end of the crash site to the other, but he was nowhere to be seen. Trying desperately to stem my panic, I realized I couldn't actually remember the last time I'd seen him.

"Blake?" I said. "Blake!" Now I struggled to move from person to person, asking if they'd seen him. My heart constricted in my chest and I couldn't think straight as I hopped at a run, calling his name.

Where could he be? He wouldn't have tried going into a burning car?

I wasn't far from hysteria now, and then I remembered Prince, all alone in the trailer, with the smells, the sounds. I bolted for Blake's truck as the scream of sirens came closer, and flashing lights heralded the arrival of the fire trucks and ambulances. I stopped when I got to the trailer to get my breath and some sort of calmness, then spoke softly to Prince through the side door. At the continued silence, I peeked inside. Standing like a rock, his nose against Blake's face, the stallion stood guard, his ears laid flat back and nostrils flaring with every breath.

22

Blake was curled up in a fetal position in front of the horse's forelegs, shaking and mumbling.

"Prince, will you let me come in?"

The stallion's ears slowly slid forward and he reached his muzzle toward me and whuffled softly as I climbed in, my ankle screaming with the effort.

I stroked his muzzle and he lipped at my fingers and I inched toward Blake. I slowly reached a hand toward Blake's shoulder, then froze, remembering Mark and the chopper. Backing up a step, I softly called out his name. He flinched, then took a breath.

"Blake, are you okay?" A little louder.

He nodded briefly, then reached a hand out to me. I took it and gripped it for all I was worth, dropped carefully to my knees and wrapped my arms around him while Prince nuzzled my hair.

"Can you tell me?" I whispered.

He shook his head, silent.

"What is it?"

"Too many memories." He shivered.

"About what?"

"Like I told you before, you'd never understand."

"I love you. Try me."

He remained motionless for long moments. "Okay, okay, I'll tell you."

I squeezed him tight, but he straightened up and I released him.

His voice was soft, nearly inaudible, and cracked as he spoke. "I was in Nam too, like Mark at the ride where we met… but I flew soldiers from the USA to Viet Nam and back with Pan Am. Many, many trips. We flew soldiers from there to R & R over the next many years—to Australia, the islands… you name it. We flew them, these men, boys, to their deaths. We flew some there and brought only some back… some in"—he swallowed hard—"in bags, or covered with bandages over missing body parts, missing minds, missing sanity. What would they suffer for the rest of their lives?" He stopped and took a deep breath. "We thought we were picking up soldiers. The girls, the stewardesses, they were shocked… at the bags and the injured men, but they talked with them." He looked up at me, almost pleading. "They held their hands, gave them the love they needed so badly. For crying out loud, they were only kids…"

He broke down and I clung to him, trying not to bump his ribs.

"They were only kids," he began again, "fighting for what? In an unpopular war…. we flew men there, hundreds at a time, and half of them were dead by the time they got back… if they went home at all."

"You did what you could," I tried again.

He went on like he hadn't heard me. "I was flying on that mercy mission Mark told us about at the ride, you know"—he glanced up at me for a moment then dropped his eyes again —"when I met you. We flew one last trip in after the airports were closed, no tower, crashed planes on the runway, you name it... to rescue the airlines' personnel from Saigon. Pan Am had promised, so along with a few volunteer air hostesses, wonderful girls... we did it."

I hugged him closer.

"But the futility... the futility of the struggle, and afterward, what did those boys, the ones who got to come home, what did they come home to? After that war, there was no respect for being one of the ones left living. Hell, it makes no sense, no sense..." His voice faded off and he lay limp in my arms, finally out of fuel.

I held him for long minutes, trying to breathe my soul into him to comfort him.

I needed to get him and the horse home.

"The ambulances are here, Blake," I whispered into his hair.

He took a deep breath and picked up his head with a wince.

The emergency services vehicles were everywhere. He struggled to a sitting position and leaned back against the wall of the trailer. Together we watched out the trailer side door as the firemen and EMTs did their jobs, and the volunteer motorists slowly filtered out, amidst thanks from the firemen. The screams quieted down to nothing as the traffic began to pass them, slowly resuming its dull roar.

Prince shuffled his feet a little, but otherwise never moved as we finished talking, wrapped in each other's arms.

Blake blinked. "We've got to go. You'll miss your plane."

"My plane." I stared at him. "If you think I'm leaving you at a time like this, you've got another thing coming. I'll get another flight."

"But—"

"No buts about it," I said, and let him painfully turn over onto all fours and stand, holding onto my hands.

We both wrapped our arms around the stallion's neck for a moment and climbed out.

"Oh my god, the place looks like a battlefield," Blake whispered and hunched up again, hugging his arms tightly to his body as a tow truck drove past us and stopped.

"Come on," I said, and walked him forward to the truck.

"What are you doing?" he said, looking at me with blank eyes as I handed him into the passenger seat of his own truck.

"I'm driving," I said, and hopped into the other side. "And you"—I pulled him over into the middle and strapped him in—"are going to sleep on my lap."

It didn't take long.

THE HOUSE WAS LIT up like a Christmas tree when we drove up the driveway. Myrtle appeared in the open doorway, while Prince's muffled and Tessa's shrill neighs filled the night.

"I heard you guys won, but where have you been? I was starting to get worried! Everyone else drove past with their trailers hours ago." The dogs scurried around our feet for a few minutes, then went off to look for rats in the barn.

"Thanks. Long story, Myrtle," I whispered. "Can you get him into bed? I've got to get Prince out and bandage him, then I'll be up, too."

Blake lifted his head. "I'm helping with the horse." His voice was hoarse. "You're in no condition—"

"Neither are you," I retorted.

"We'll do it together," he said, and I didn't have the strength to argue. My leg was throbbing again.

"Why are you limping?" Myrtle peered at my face in the dimness.

"That's a long story, too," I said.

Myrtle shook her head. "Everybody's been fed, and I'll

draw you both a bath," she said. Turning on her heel, she headed back to the house. "Come on, dogs, back to bed," she called, and they followed, looking longingly back at the barn.

"Bless you," I said, meaning it with all my heart, as I hopped to the back of the trailer and unlatched Prince's ramp. I didn't think I could take dogs bouncing off my leg tonight. Blake and I got the stallion out of the trailer and led him to his dinner in the barn. Tessa raced into her stall from her attached pen and stood staring at us over her half-door.

"You have some under-quilts and track bandages, Blake?"

He nodded.

I eased myself on a low stool, my bad leg straight out alongside the stallion and, untwisted the cap on the liniment. My tongue curled at the alcoholic menthol fumes as I rubbed a few generous handfuls onto Prince's first leg.

I cringed at the sound of clanging cupboards and swearing from the tack room but it resulted in an armload of bandaging that Blake laid out on a makeshift table of hay bales beside me.

I bandaged one leg while Blake moved on to the next with the liniment, and soon we were somehow done with them all. All the while, Prince never moved a hoof or picked up his head from his feed bucket. After greeting his mate, of course.

"He's a good horse," I said, after one last hug. "Thanks, Prince, and Blake."

Blake gave me the ghost of a smile as he wrapped an arm around me and helped me limp my way up to the house.

The answerphone was blinking red when we walked in.

"Your supper's on the table," Myrtle called from upstairs. "Let me know if I can do anything to help, otherwise, I'll hear your news in the morning. Good night."

I punched the button on the flashing machine as I took a bite of the steaming quiche Myrtle had left for us.

"This is a message for Lena Scott from the veterinary school. Lena, I called to tell you you've passed your Small

Animal Medicine rotation and are on track to graduate on time. Enjoy your last few days of vacation. Goodbye."

My eyes met Blakes and he reached for me. I closed my eyes and sank onto his lap.

"Congratulations, girl," he whispered into my hair, "on all counts, today."

As if winning the race wasn't enough.

We shared our last bites of pastry with the dogs, wished them goodnight, and then I limped towards the stairs.

Blake sighed. "Wait for me," he said. "You have to be the most impatient little brat I've ever met," he murmured, as he kissed my lips and reached out his arms to pick me up and froze.

"With broken ribs?" I couldn't help a giggle as I shook my head.

"I was going to carry you up to bed, but—"

"Thanks for the thought. Next time, maybe?" I said, and we struggled up the stairs like a couple of oldies that smelled like they hadn't bathed in weeks and tried to cover it up with liniment.

Couldn't wait to get into that tub.

"And so, Raywyn," I said into the mouthpiece of the phone, lazily lying back in a rocking chair on Blake's deck, my foot up on a box, "I wanted to thank you."

"For what? Just a sec," Ray said, and her muffled voice gave some go-home instructions on a blocked cat to the new technician. "Sorry, it's my lunch hour, but the Doc is out. Now, where were we? You wanted to thank me? For what?"

"Yes. If not for you, I wouldn't have ever met Blake."

"So, are you truly so happy?"

"I am, we are."

"And you don't think the age difference is… going to be a problem? Truly?"

"Nope. We're doing fine. Really. And he's supportive, mostly. He just misses me."

"And do you miss him?"

I was silent for a moment. "Sort of, but really, I only have time for school right now, and he understands that. We see each other when we can. That'll have to be enough for now."

"Well, if you're sure."

"I am."

"Okay, then you have my blessing. When's the wedding?"

"Sometime after I graduate, I think. We haven't planned it yet, but there won't be time until then."

"Well, I'll be there, holding your hand."

"Love ya, Ray."

"You too, Lena. You take care, okay? Congrats on the win with that stallion. I've got to go, but we'll speak soon, okay?"

"Bye, and thanks again."

The phone clicked in my ear.

It would all be okay. Jake plopped his head onto my lap and I patted him in the warm sunshine until I melted into sleep.

"YOUR JEALOUSY, though, Blake, it makes me feel you don't trust me," I said the following night as we sat on the sheepskins before a roaring fire, my bad foot elevated on the sofa. "I've given you no reason to distrust me. We've talked of this so many times before…"

"I was afraid of losing you from my life." He fell silent for a few moments. "You remember wondering how I was content to just live a quiet life, content to sit on my porch with you and the dogs, no ambitions?"

Wincing, I looked him fully in the eyes and nodded.

"Think about last night," he said. "Really think about it for a second."

I closed my eyes and shivered, remembering the carnage… the carnage on the road, and in Blake's heart. I swallowed hard. "I think I begin to see," I finally murmured. "I'm sorry, Blake, I never saw it before. The 'what's important'. I've been struggling so long to succeed—to get into vet school, and now to get *back out* of vet school… I guess everything doesn't have to be full-on, every minute, to stay on track for my dreams… and life."

"It's taken me just as long to see you're not going to disappear." Blake took my hand. "When you've seen the things I have," he stared blankly out the window into the darkness, then turned back to me, "you're thankful for the life you've created and the special animals and people you've been given. Like you." He sat in silence for a moment. "I'm willing to give you the time and space you need to complete your lifelong dream, and I want to be there beside you to share the finis—"

At a knock upon the door, the dogs set up a cacophony as they raced toward it and flung themselves against the groaning wood.

"Whoever could it be at this hour?" I stared at Blake.

He climbed to his feet and grabbed Kelpie Anne's collar, then opened the door.

In the doorway stood Seth Latimer.

"Come on in, man, what are you doing out at this hour?"

"Thanks," Doc Latimer said, as he swept his hat off and hung it on the hat rack. He came over and sat down on the sofa across from me. "I saw your lights on and figured you were still awake."

"Like the welcoming committee would've let us sleep through that," I said dryly, then laughed.

Seth grinned at me. "I'm on my way home from a colic

and wanted to see how that ankle was. I see you're behaving, Lena." He nodded approvingly at my raised foot.

"It's good, thanks. They said it was a sprain, but they want to x-ray it again in a few weeks to make sure there aren't any fractures. It's a little swollen."

With a growl beneath his breath, Seth said, "What a surprise, after riding with it like that for half of the ride, or so…"

"I took my feet out of my stirrups…" I twisted my lips and shrugged.

"Probably because you couldn't *ride* in stirrups, you cretin," Blake muttered.

"Well, it was splinted."

"What about elevated?"

"Children, children…" Seth said, "I also wanted to let you know I read the riot act to our good Dr. Barnett-Payne and put in a formal complaint to the Veterinary Medical Board. I told him, but it doesn't seem to register that it's not someone else's fault." He shook his head. "Never seen anything like it."

"He's a special one, all right," I mumbled. "I was a bit slow to learn his true nature."

"Good thing you figured it out," Seth said, nodding. "Anyway, I'm sorry for the difficulties he's caused and I wanted to congratulate you again on your win, but especially on your Best Condition award."

"Thanks," I said, "but it's Blake who conditioned that horse. It should by rights be his."

Seth stood, then faced me with a smile. "We really do need an equine vet up in this valley. Goodnight to you both," he said as he walked out the door into the chilly night.

After he closed the door behind the good doctor, Blake carefully lowered his sore body down to the sheepskins again, only wincing a little, and looked into my eyes. "I'd say, compared to the past two days, the chances of you and I making a serious go of it will be easy as pie."

I smiled at him and sniffed. "What's that smell?" I asked as the sickly-sweet scent of burning sugar invaded my nostrils. "Something's burning."

"Thought we both deserved something special." He winked at me. "While you were napping, I went to the bakery."

"Cherry pie!"

Blake's smile lit his whole face and I stretched up to kiss his lips, then he groaned as he pulled himself up to full height once again and headed off to save the pie.

Life would be good, together.

The End

Thank you for joining Lena and Kit in
Fifty Miles at a Breath.
Lena will be returning in other books in the series.

Enjoyed the story? Want to read more?
*If you loved it, a short review on Bookbub, Goodreads and your favorite eBook retailer would sure be appreciated.
I'd be grateful for your help in spreading the word!*

Sign up for Lizzi's VIP Readers Club to hear about new releases and specials, plus get your free sampler gift here:

www.lizzitremayne.com/VIP50

FIND BOOKS

Find eBooks at your favorite online retailer via buy links at www.lizzitremayne.com

or

Purchase Softcover books:

from New Zealand and Australia,

My print books are available in standard (and some in large format) print for your reading pleasure. Find bookstores stocking my books at:

www.lizzitremayne.com/Booksellers

From Other Countries:

Print books are available in paperback from most online retailers and in select bookstores around the world.

Find stockists at www.lizzitremayne.com/Booksellers

BOOKS BY THE AUTHOR

The Long Trails Series

Books 1-3: ***The Long Trails Box Set: Historical Western Family Saga: Books 1-3***

Can an orphan, with only her Mustang and a Cossack sword, survive alone on the frontier?

From the deserts of Utah, through the gold mines of California, to the turbulent wilderness of Colonial New Zealand, Aleksandra rides, loves, and fights—with only her Cossack skills to keep her alive.

Book One: ***A Long Trail Rolling***

Winner of the True West Magazine 2016 Best Western Romance, Winner Romance Writers of New Zealand: 2014 Pacific Hearts Award and 2015 Koru Award

Hunted for her secrets. Hiding in plain sight. Can one woman blaze her own trail into untamed territory?

UTAH TERRITORY, 1860. Aleksandra has spent her whole life training for the inevitable. So, when a brutal Cossack tracks down and kills her father, she instinctively collects her pa's elixir and flees. But when she meets the mysterious Xavier at a nearby trading post, she wonders if she can win both his protection and his heart…

Disappointed when the man of her dreams leaves to join the Pony Express, Aleksandra dons a disguise to follow him into the dangerous frontier assignment. Hiding behind her martial arts skills and a male alias, she longs to tell the handsome Xavier the truth. But with the killer in pursuit, keeping up the ruse may be her only chance for survival…

Can Aleksandra save both her love and her family legacy from a relentless murderer?

Book Two: *The Hills of Gold Unchanging*

As the Civil War rages, secessionists menace California. The Confederates want the state and they'll stop at nothing to take it.

UTAH TERRITORY, 1860. On a wagon train headed West, Aleksandra makes an enemy of a gun-running Confederate when she fights her way out of his unwelcome embrace and Xavier's new friends realize he's heard too much to be allowed to live. Embroiled in the Confederate's fight to drag the new state from the Union and make it their own, can Aleks and Xavier survive? The secessionists mean business.

Book Three: *A Sea of Green Unfolding*

They set sail for the peace and calm of New Zealand, but they hadn't counted on murderers, mutineers, and a land war in paradise.

SAN FRANCISCO BAY AND NEW ZEALAND, 1863. Tragedy strikes in Aleksandra and Xavier's newly found paradise on their California Rancho but Von Tempsky's invitation draws them to a new life in peaceful New Zealand. They disembark into a turbulent wilderness—with the opening shots of the New Zealand Wars just being fired—straight at them.

Novella: **Somewhere Called Home**

Highlands to Waterloo—can love prevail over fate?

SCOTTISH HIGHLANDS, 1813.

Robert is disowned for refusing to become clan tacksman after his father and heads for the city, alone, to build a life for himself and his beloved Sofia. Sofia's waiting turns to despair when her mother buys safety during the clearance of their village—leaving Sofia at the mercy of the laird's degenerate son. Rob emerges from the hell of Waterloo wanting only to see Sofia again... and his father. *To be released soon.*

The *Tatiana* Series
(with links to The Long Trails *series)*

Book One: **Tatiana I**

Stableman's daughter Tatiana rises to glamorous heights by her equestrienne abilities—but the tsar's glittering attention is not always gold.

MOSKVA, RUSSIA 1842. Tatiana and her husband Vladimir become pawns in the emperor's pursuit of a coveted secret weapon. While Tatiana and their infant son are placed under house arrest, Vladimir must recover the weapon or lose his wife and young son. With the odds mounting against them, can they find each other again—half a world away? *Coming soon!*

The Once Upon a Vet School Series

Drama and humor abound as Lena pursues her childhood dream of becoming an equine vet—and beyond—in this unique series of

six independent novella sequences:

~Junior Years~

After Lena hears she needs good grades to become a veterinarian, things start to get tricky. Even her pony doesn't get out unscathed. (Middle Grade) **USA 1972-1976**

~High School Days ~

When your high school counsellor says vet school's too hard for you and your HS sweetheart offers you a dream life of farming, writing, and babies, what do you do? Is vet school really the be-all, end-all? (Young Adult) ***USA 1976-1979***

~College Nights~

How can you have a life when you need an A in every class for four years to get into vet school... on top of 800 hours vet practice work? Something's got to give. (Young Adult and up) ***USA 1980-1984***

~Vet School 24/7~

Now they're in, the pressure for grades is off and vet school social life is upon them... there's only the tsunami of 200 years of veterinary knowledge to pack into their heads. Can Lena and her friends stay afloat? (Young Adult and up) ***USA 1984-1988***

~Practice Time~

Finally graduated, prima ballerinas of the university, Lena and her vet school classmates disperse to far-flung practices... and real life. What could possibly go wrong? Late nights on-call, mud, blood, and finally, a light at the end of the tunnel... unfortunately, it's only the penlight of a dictatorial vet technician in Lena's eyes after she passed out on the floor. (Women's Rural Fiction with Romantic Elements) ***USA & New Zealand 1988-2012***

~Long in the Tooth~

When Lena suffers another catastrophic back injury in New Zealand, what's she to do to feed her family and keep the farm? She can't breathe around cats or birds and what good's an equine vet who can't hold up a horse's leg? Time for Lena to go back to school. Again. (Women's Rural Fiction with Romantic Elements) ***New Zealand 2012- ...***

Currently Available Reads:
~Vet School 24/7~

Fifty Miles at a Breath

Horses bring them together and their future looks rosy—it's the present they can't handle.

When equine veterinary student Lena and veteran pilot Blake fall in love, vet school and the past intrude. Add in a long-distance relationship, and things get just plain hard. A grueling endurance race forces them to draw on their strengths and face their fears —together.

Lena Takes a Foal

She needs help... he needs to stay away...

Lena's got a problem—one that might prevent her from graduating. When her horse flips over and lands on her, it has to be the dashing resident, Kit, who finds her. Luckily, she's sworn off relationships after her last debacle and sea-green eyes and rugged good looks are the last things on her mind. Besides, to a veterinary school faculty, relationships between residents and students are like oil and water.

They just don't mix.

~Practice Time~

Greener Pastures Calling

A new country, a great job, and a good Kiwi bloke. Life couldn't be better.

Until it gets worse.

Newly emigrated to New Zealand, Lena wants a 'good Kiwi bloke', but they're elusive as their nocturnal namesake. Nigel's avoiding females, unless they're cows, horses, or his mother after his first marriage. Sparks fly when they meet—but not the first time, over the dirty instruments in a filthy cowshed. They seem to be made for each other, until Nigel remembers where he first saw her. And then the questions start.

Understanding Modern Vet Med for Owners

The new series of veterinary books for horse owners to let you use what vets know to keep your horses healthier and happier. *First volume due out soon!*

With Bluestocking Belles

Boxed sets of historical love stories from a host of bestselling authors.

Christmas 2018: *Follow Your Star Home*

The Viking star ring is said to bring lovers together, no matter how far, no matter how hard.

In nine stories, covering more than half the world and a thousand years, our heroes and heroines put the legend to the test. Watch the star work its magic, as prodigals return home in the season of good will, uncertain of their welcome.

With Authors of Main Street

Boxed sets of *new* contemporary love stories from multiple bestselling authors, for a sweet romantic holiday treat.

Christmas 2017: *Christmas Babies on Main Street Nine stories from the bestselling Authors of Main Street!*

From the small hamlet of Eastport, to the gorgeous landscapes of New Zealand, to Main Street, USA, you'll find the Christmas spirit and warm love stories on every page.

Summer 2018: *Summer Romance on Main Street*

Seven stories from the Authors of Main Street!

Welcome to Main Street, where you'll find sweet summer romance and true love from small towns everywhere

Christmas 2018: *Christmas Wishes on Main Street*

Seven stories from the Authors of Main Street

Don't you love to hear everyone's Christmas wishes? Read our small town wishes and feel the love from Canada all the way through to New Zealand.

Sign up for Lizzi's VIP Reader Club to hear about new releases and specials, plus get your free sampler gift here!

www.lizzitremayne.com/VIP50

Lizzi Tremayne's Books
2019

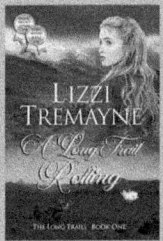
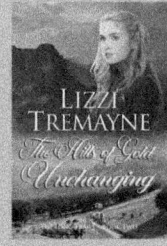
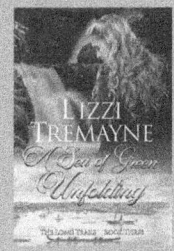
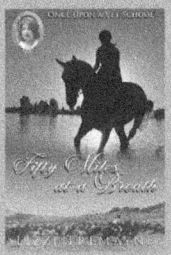
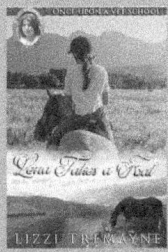
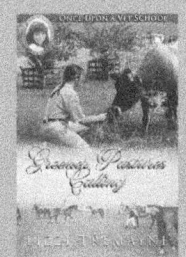

Coming Soon!

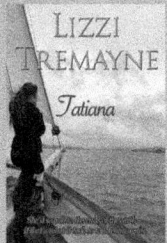
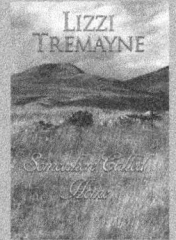

With Love from
New Zealand, Russia, Scotland, and U.S.A.

AUTHOR'S NOTES

On the off chance that you haven't figured it out by now, much of this story is based upon my life and times during veterinary school.

I grew up in an "endurance family" as Lena did in the story. I've ridden in endurance races and ride & ties (even the Levi Ride & Tie!) and vetted rides in California and Nevada. I have the utmost respect for the team of riders, crews, and veterinarians who keep these splendid horses safe. A rider has the choice of whether or not to go on, but the horse does not. It's up to the *whole team* to ensure they're not overfaced and endangered.

The incident in the story with the exhausted horse, sadly, is drawn from a past experience when I was vetting. The biggest difference? The actual patient was in worse shape than Sabado, but fortunately it's rare these days. Thankfully for the horses, AERC, the American Endurance Ride Conference, does a fantastic job of helping riders gain access the information they need to take the very best care of their horses. Thanks, AERC!

I hope you enjoy your foray into my world of veterinary fiction. If you liked it, help others find it by leaving reviews and comments where you purchased it, on Bookbub, Goodreads, and on my webpage. If you want to pass on a comment, please find me via my *Connect with Lizzi* page.

Warmest regards,

Lizzi Tremayne

RECIPE: COTTAGE CHEESE PANCAKES

Lena and I love both of these high protein, quick, healthy, and yummy pancakes. You can make them with oats or wheat.

Cottage Cheese Pancakes with Flour (2 moderate servings. Double this for two hungry teenagers and you.)

- 3 eggs
- 1 c (250 g) cottage cheese
- 2 T (30 ml) Oil
- 1/4 c (30 g) flour

Cottage Cheese Pancakes with Oats—GF* (2 large servings)

- 7 large or 8 smaller eggs
- 1 c (250 g) cottage cheese
- 1 c (100 g) rolled oats, uncooked

Instructions for either recipe:
1- Break eggs into bowl or blender *first*, then add cottage

cheese. Blend in a blender, food processor, or with a stick blender. Alternately, whisk or beat them with a spoon.

2- Add the other ingredients and mix until smooth—as little or as much as you like.

3- Using about 1/4 c (60 ml) batter per pancake, fry in a hot pan or on the hot flat plate of a barbecue (we use our barbecue) with a little butter, oil, or drippings over a medium heat.

4- Turn when bubbles appear, then cook until both sides are golden.

NB: The pancakes from the first recipe stick together a bit better, in case that matters to you.

Serve with:

Applesauce, cooked up fruit (great way to use up overripe fruit), fruit syrup, bananas, yogurt or sour cream, maple syrup, honey… you name it.

Our favorite here is to drop banana slices into the just-poured batter. If mum isn't looking, the boys add chocolate chips at the same time.

Bon appétit!

*Oats themselves are gluten free but check the label in case gluten-containing products are made on same equipment.

ABOUT THE AUTHOR

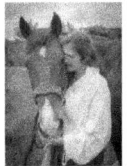

Lizzi grew up riding wild in the Santa Cruz Mountain redwoods, became an equine veterinarian at UC Davis School of Veterinary Medicine and practiced in the Gold and Pony Express Country of California before emigrating to New Zealand. She has two wonderful boys, a grandbaby, and an awesome partner in that sea of green. When she's not writing, she's swinging a rapier or shooting a bow in medieval garb, riding or driving a carriage, playing in the garden on her hobby farm, singing, cooking, or looking into a horse's mouth in her equine veterinary dental practice. She is multiply published and awarded in special interest magazines and veterinary periodicals.

With this debut novel, she was Finalist 2013 RWNZ Great Beginnings, Winner 2014 RWNZ Pacific Hearts Award for the unpublished full manuscript, Winner 2015 RWNZ Koru Award for Best First Novel and third in Koru Long Novel, and Finalist 2015 Best Indie Book Award.

CONNECT WITH LIZZI

I'm looking forward to hearing from you!

Join conversations and find story excerpts, buy links, and more here:

www.lizzitremayne.com/VIP50
www.lizzitremayne.com
www.horseandvetbooks.com
www.bookandmainbites.com/LizziTremayne/
www.bookbub.com/profile/lizzi-tremayne/
www.facebook.com/lizzitremayneauthor/
www.instagram.com/lizzitremayne/
www.twitter.com/LizziTremayne/
www.youtube.com/user/lizzikiwi/
www.goodreads.com/LizziTremayne/
https://nz.pinterest.com/lizzitremayne/

ACKNOWLEDGMENTS

To Bob~
Thank you for all the smiles, the encouragement, and the caring. RIP. xx

To Matthew~
I've said this before and I'll say it again. As you keep saying, I may be doing the writing, publishing, promo, and the everything else to get my stories out there… but I couldn't do it without your support, love, and care. Yes, I could do it on my own, but I'd be just as 24/7-frazzled as I once was. (Sorry to my boys. xx) Thank you from the bottom of my heart for making my life not only reasonable, but exquisite. xx

To my Wonderful Beta Readers, Kirsten Davidson, Marjorie Jones, Jude Knight, Kate Le Petit, Matthew Mole, and last but not least, Sharon Smith~
Without you, this story would have been just the one-eyed blather than comes out of my pen sometimes. And at short notice. You're all gold. Thank you so much. xx

EXCERPT FROM A LONG TRAIL ROLLING

April 1860, Echo Canyon, Utah Territory, U.S.A.

SHE SMELLED BLOOD. Its metallic tang assailed her senses before it was overshadowed by the stench of death. Stepping back to scan the sheer wall of the bluff rising before her, her breath caught in her throat and a sob escaped.

Finally, she'd found him.

A scuffed black boot and fur coat showed through the snow, his body wedged into the bottom of a crevice three feet above her head. She looked up to the top of the cliff, from which he must have fallen, but saw no one.

Finding handholds where there were none, Aleksandra Lekarski scrambled up the wall as her heart constricted in her chest. She tugged her father's cold, stiff body free and down onto level ground, giving thanks he'd been out of reach of the wolves whose tracks abounded in the snow where she now stood. Her world blurred as she dropped to her knees and cradled his lifeless head in her lap, rocking him. Ceaseless tears flowed down her doeskin tunic.

With a numbing pain in her mind, she ran shaking hands over him, seeking answers. What could have made an experienced trapper like Krzysztof Lekarski fall off a bluff and succumb to a death more suited to a greenhorn?

This couldn't really be happening.

Just seven days ago, he'd kissed her goodbye with glowing eyes.

'Keep the fire going in the smokehouse this time, will you, Aleks?'

'Of course, Papa, my promise. Be back soon, I'll miss you.'

'I'll return before you've missed me, then we'll go sell last winter's furs at the trading post.'

We'll never go to town together again.

Aleksandra sat back on her heels and gripped her swimming head in her hands, fingers pulling her hair until it hurt, then whimpered and returned her attention to her papa.

She shrank from what was left of his eyes… and was glad he'd been in the narrow gap, too small for large predators. Beetles had been there, or some rodent, maybe even a hawk. The scent of decay was a sharp contrast to the clean bite of fresh snow. Trying not to breathe through her nose, she swallowed hard, stomach rolling.

Aleksandra's hands froze as hard-crusted blood met her fingertips. Her heart stopped altogether at the sight of the inch-long, bloodied cut in his buckskin jerkin, repeating into his chest wall. She turned him over. A laceration of the same size exited the soft leather covering his back.

Papa hadn't simply fallen off the bluff. Nothing but a sword made such a wound.

Aleksandra's ears began to ring, her world narrowing to a small gap, as she fought the rising panic.

It couldn't be...Vladimir couldn't *have found us. Not over two decades, two continents and the Atlantic Ocean.*

The ground swayed as she hunched over her father's still form. Squeezing her eyes shut to stop the motion, she recalled the words Papa had endlessly repeated, so she would always remember:

'He *will* seek us out. Vladimir will come for the secret and we must be prepared to keep it from him—at all costs —always.'

But what a cost.

Despite her entire being screaming to fall apart for the loss of her only remaining family, years of Papa's training to protect their secret stopped her in her tracks. Struggling to draw air into her lungs, she looked around the bottom of the cliff. Her clearing vision now showed more wolf sign: scrapings on the wall below his body and white snow darkened by blood beside stinking yellow patches.

Leaving his body here, knowing the scavengers would return, would be the hardest thing she'd ever done—but Aleksandra knew what her papa would have required of her.

Heart sinking, she slumped to the forest floor beside him and took a deep breath of the wind whistling cold up the valley. Closing her eyes, she touched her lips to the top of his head. With shaking hands and tears flowing anew, Aleksandra lifted the leather thong of the beaded *Shoshone* medicine bag from about his neck and pulled the signet ring from his finger. Kissing her papa once more, she covered him with dead leaves and snow, beseeching the forest spirits to care for him with love, if she couldn't return.

She rose and turned to leave, but through the brain-fogging misery, she remembered to check for the tools of Papa's trade. The trapper's sword scabbard was empty and his rifle missing. The firearm was nearby, half covered by a snowy branch, but even after searching for precious minutes, his *shashka* was nowhere to be found. With a twinge of regret, she gave up seeking her father's Cossack sword. She shouldered the rifle and stared back at the man she loved beyond life, her heart in a vise, with a promise and a prayer for his soul. Tears dried cold and tight on her face as she stood gazing past the putrefying corpse to the heart of her papa. She returned once more to brush back the frozen leaves and kiss him goodbye.

Her eyes scanned the aspen glade in the brilliant morning light. No one watched. With the silence and speed of the *kwahaten*, the antelope, her name with the *Shoshone* people who had welcomed her family into their own, she ran for her pony.

'It's you and me now, Dzień,' she choked out as she untied him and slung the rifle on her back. Vaulting on as he struck off into a lope, they flew back toward the cabin, the Indian pony seeming to sense the urgency and single-mindedness of his mistress. Slowing him to a stealthy walk as they neared the cabin, she slid from Dzień's back, signaling him to wait. She crept closer to the cabin. Before its open door, papers lay scattered beneath a light dusting of snow, fluttering in the chill breeze. The open barn doors slowly swung back and forth.

By now Papa's stallion should have been tearing up the stable and his field, but Rogan was gone. She waited, straining every muscle for any sound, but only silence met her ears, save the creaking hinges. She tiptoed around the perimeter of the yard in soft deerskin moccasins, keeping to the tree shadows as she'd done with her *Shoshone* friends in play. Hidden in shadow, Aleksandra stole to the window at the back of the cabin and peered in.

Her breath caught at the destruction. An intruder had turned the cabin upside down and must have set-to the place with a sword. The white softness of sliced feather-tick mattresses covered every surface and bedclothes were ribboned and strewn over the floorboards, but there was no movement.

She eased the door open and slid inside, hand on the hilt of her own *shashka*.

The doors of the oak secretary, Krzysztof's gift to Aleksandra's mother just before her death two winters ago, lay open. She nearly cried to see its drawers flung helter-skelter and papers scattered.

Utensils danced amongst broken crockery and cast iron pans. In some dim recess of her mind, she noticed the *zakwas* and sourdough pots still stood on their shelf behind the cook stove, high above the chaos.

She broke into a sweat at the sight of the stove lids lying in deep, black grooves in the wooden floor of the cabin. Lids hot enough to burn themselves into the cedar planks meant she'd narrowly missed the visit of the intruder when she left the cabin to find her pa.

She froze. Nothing of value seemed to be missing. This was only a search. Her heart sank further at the sight of the sun-bleached muslin dress on its peg in the corner by her bed, doubtless informing the unwelcome visitor, by now almost certainly the Russian Vladimir, that someone besides Krzysztof lived here.

Aleksandra climbed onto the table and peered up into the eaves. Papa's velvet-lined boxes were still in their places. She lifted the lids and nearly smiled, then hopped down and slipped out the door. Skirting the yard again, she noiselessly opened the back door of the barn and peeked in. The summer smell of new hay assailed her nostrils as she entered and surveyed the damage. The trespasser had been busy here too.

Harnesses and building tools were scattered about the dirt floor, the contents of the feed room and hay pile scattered.

Well, that accounts for the scent.

The buckboard wagon and dogcart were still there, but the gate rails of Rogan's loosebox lay where they'd been dropped. The manure in the stall was dry, several days old.

She glanced around the darkened corners of the barn and the yard outside once more before returning to squeeze her hand into the secret cache behind the colt's feed bin. As her fingers chilled at the touch of the dozen or so frigid glass vials and the box next to it, her lips twisted into a bittersweet smile. For the first time in days, the leaden melancholy lifted from her shoulders, if only a little. Despite the destruction, Vladimir had missed what he came for.

What now? Aleksandra ruminated, shaking her head, then took a great lungful of air.

Dzień trotted up at her whistle and she resolutely wiped her tears onto his mane, then hugged him around the neck with the hint of a smile.

'Papa's secret is safe, Dzień. We can bring him home,' she murmured, pressing her face into his furry neck. Reaching around, he nuzzled her derriere in reply and Aleksandra twisted to kiss him on his white star. She pulled the bedroll and bags from her saddle, then led him to the travois just inside the barn. She adjusted the two long poles, bound together with woven rawhide strips, then covered the widest part of the litter with a buffalo rug. Her papa's conveyance was complete.

On the long walk back to the bluff, she thought of her father's loving touch, his constant presence in her life, his sweet smile, his twinkling eyes. She would have them no more. Spiraling downward again, the thought of drowning in the emptiness was almost welcome, but she gritted her teeth and mentally shook herself. The focus was now on survival. Aleksandra suspected Vladimir didn't know the exact nature of what he sought, but nonetheless, he would return. She needed to be ready. Better yet, gone.

Aleksandra didn't fool herself. Her father, a survivor of Austro-Hungarian-occupied Poland, spent countless hours teaching his children self-defense. Unfortunately, Aleksandra's skills with a *shashka* were a fraction of those of her papa's... and even less than those of *his* own teacher, Vladimir. The Russian was, according to Papa, unsurpassed with the short Russian Cossack sword.

'You're a good swordsman, Aleks, but your impetuosity gets you into trouble,' Papa always said, shaking his head as he disarmed her, yet again. The last time, he'd added: '...whether you're sparring at *shashkas* or trying to knit for the memory of your mama, God rest her soul, who tried to reconcile you to your femaleness.'

Aleksandra grinned through her tears. Knitting that always ended up as a wad of uneven and dropped stitches—inevitably thrown in fit of temper onto a set of antlers high upon the sitting room wall.

ROUNDING the bottom of the bluff, Dzień picked up his head and pricked his ears, sniffing the breeze, then headed for the pile of leaves covering Krzysztof. He stopped dead six feet away.

Aleksandra gave him a pat on the neck and tried to smile, but failed. She left the pony's head to adjust the travois. Breathing deeply through flared nostrils, Dzień stepped towards Krzysztof. He shook his mane, then nuzzled the lifeless body, knocking off the leaves as he checked the man's full length. Dzień tapped him with a front hoof, then snorted and turned away, showing the whites of his eyes as he stared at the motionless man from the corner of one eye. Aleksandra's gut wrenched.

Blood pounded in her head as she struggled to drag Krzysztof's six-foot frame onto the makeshift stretcher. Dzień craned his neck around to watch, his muzzle and the skin about his eyes tensed and strained.

The pony responded to Aleksandra's gentle urging and took Krzysztof home one last time. She would bury him with his beloved wife and sons in their overpopulated graveyard, then determine how to elude Vladimir and survive.

'Can't protect our secret if you're dead, *moje drogie córki.*' Papa's words came back to her, in his thickly accented but precise English.

"*My darling daughter.*" Gulping, she clutched her father's medicine bag and choked back more tears, realizing she'd never hear those words again.

Sign up for Lizzi's VIP Reader Club to hear about new releases and specials, plus get your free sampler gift at www.lizzitremayne/VIP50

EXCERPT FROM TATIANA

M*id-1842 Moskva, Russia*

BY THE TIME I was fifteen, and Vladimir sixteen, we were inseparable. No longer did he clean stalls as punishment, but to help me before his Training School classes began. This gave us more time to fit ourselves and prepare our combined *džigitovka* performances. We had been selected as part of the team to perform for the Tsar on his next visit to Moskva from St. Petersburg.

The tsar's creepy messenger, who came to our door with increasing regularity for no seemingly good reason, had delivered the invitation for our group to give the performance. His terse smile showed through the lace curtains as he stood before the door. I managed to talk Papa into answering it, claiming I couldn't leave my cooking pot.

The messenger, whose name I never asked, but he told me anyway, was Sambor Andropov. Due to his frequent visits, I had taken to ignoring anyone knocking on the door when I was in the house alone. His mere eyes on me made my skin crawl, and I felt I was being undressed before his eyes. Although a servant of the tsar could not be ignored without serious repercussion, if he didn't know I was there, all would be well. If the message was important, he would return, or Mrs. Bagrov would get the door if she was in.

I had the grace to be embarrassed when I realized he had carried such a special invitation to our door after I had avoided him. It was just that men and boys in Papa stableyard never looked at me like that, so perhaps I was being overly sensitive. I vowed to be kinder to him when I saw him next. He was, after all, just doing the tsar's bidding.

After this missive, our training intensified. We only had a month to prepare our troop for our presentation before Tsar Nicholas and his Empress Alexsandra Feodorovna.

There were eleven men in our group, plus me. We were drawn from the wider area around Moskva, but bragging aside, Vladimir and I were the stars of the show.

We had a joint act, with a quadrangle, jumping and shashka work, but our own little act was the best one. It began with Vladimir and I standing in Sarda's saddle, with me just behind him, one hand in the air, waving at the audience. We would then do a lift, ending up with my standing upon Vladimir's shoulders—at a full gallop.

It was a truly tricky maneuver, and one that few ever attempted. We lived, ate and breathed *džigitovka*. In any spare time, we worked out together— running, press-ups, sit-ups— we needed all the strength we could muster, and on the day of the performance for the Tsar Nicholas and Tsarina Alexandra Feodorovna, we triumphed.

During our bows to their Excellencies, the Empress Alexandra Feodorovna beckoned us closer.

"Your skills," she said, "for such young people are to be rewarded. I should like to see you both again." She paused for a moment. "Perhaps," she glanced at the tsar, who lifted an eyebrow at her, and then turned back to us, "you would like to attend the ball at the Kremlin tomorrow night?"

I swallowed hard.

"We should be honored, your Excellencies," Vladimir said, his voice smooth.

"We will see you there." The tsarina nodded and turned back toward her husband, dismissing us.

I curtsied as gracefully as I could, holding a pair of reins and wearing jodhpurs and boots, lacking the essential skirts. Vladimir drew me to my feet and escorted me away.

"A ball at the Kremlin?" I blinked and took a deep breath. "However will I find a ball dress before tomorrow night?"

"You have none?" He looked at me, jaw dropped.

I peered from beneath my brows. "How many balls have I attended since we met?"

He stared at me. "Well…"

"Exactly. I attended the end of year cadets ball with you last year, but that dress will hardly be suitable for an audience," I indicated my breeches and boots, "other than this, of course, with the tsar and tsarina. It's easy for you. You simply need your Training School dress uniform."

"Sisters. Yes, that's it." He spun to face me. "Olga and Sonja will have a dress to fit you."

My jaw dropped. His sisters were elegant young ladies. I'd been introduced to them before, but they hadn't seemed impressed by the stable girl performing with their brother. "But they live a full day's ride away. I'd never be able to ride there and return and still take care of my stable duties."

"I'll go. I can get one of the other lads to do my work for me, if your father permits."

"I permit," he said, walking up in time to hear the end of the conversation.

"Thank you, sir. I have three sisters, most of them close in size to Tatiana. With your permission, I will leave as soon as I cool out my horse."

"We'll take care of that and inform the headmaster. Well done, both of you. Your performance was without equal," he said, taking the reins of Vladimir's horse and leading him back toward the barn.

"Papa," I said, and he turned. I reached out for Sarda's reins. "Thank you, for all you've done for me, for us." I glanced at Vladimir's retreating back.

He handed them to me and hugged me, his eyes glistening with unshed tears. "You have made me so proud, both you and Vladimir. What a team you make."

"We could've never done it without you."

"Soon he will be finished here and must enter the tsar's army." He took back Sarda's reins and together we began walking the sweating horses. "Have you considered what you will do then?" His eyes looked at me—through me—and I shuddered, then swallowed and looked at the floor.

"I honestly do not know, Papa."

"A life of horses is hard for a man, much less a woman, and I won't be around forever."

My eyes snapped up to his. "What?" For the first time, I saw his weathered visage, the grayness of his skin at the edges, and my stomach clenched. "Papa, are you ill?"

He took a deep breath. "I'm not sure, but my heart, it does funny things sometimes. Not badly, but it's enough to give me pause—to question and to ensure you are provided for."

The walls of the Kremlin swayed around me. Papa was my rock, although I'd been increasingly leaning on Vladimir as we had become close friends, and now, it seems, something more.

"Have you been to a doctor, Papa?" Knowing her hadn't.

"No, but there is little they could do."

"You don't know that…"

"Trust me, I know. Anyway, *princessa*, you will be going to the ball and dancing the night away on the arm of your prince.

"Will you becoming?"

"The invitation was only for the two of you, but I will be awaiting your return with bated breath." I offered the horse a few sips of water from a bucket then pulled Sarda away and we resumed our walk.

"This will be my first ball without you, Papa…" I searched his face, seeking to know the extent of his sickness, but nothing showed.

"My *solnishko* has grown up." New tears in his eyes threatened to fall. "You will be the loveliest woman there."

Woman.

I'd never thought of myself as that…it would take some time to sink in.

Due out soon! Look for it!

Sign up for Lizzi's VIP Reader Club to hear about new releases and specials, plus get your free sampler gift at
www.lizzitremayne/VIP50

*Thank you for reading.
I hope you enjoyed Fifty Miles at a Breath!*

*Sign up to join Lizzi's VIP Reader Club and hear about new release and specials, plus get your free book!
It's right here:*

www.lizzitremayne/VIP50

www.ingramcontent.com/pod-product-compliance
Lightning Source LLC
Chambersburg PA
CBHW070118100426
42744CB00010B/1861